"An invaluable resource for clinicians and other practitioners dealing with the impacts of substance use"

Olaf H. Drummer, *Professor Emeritus, Victorian Institute of Forensic Medicine and Monash University*

"Already a core text in clinical forensic medicine this book is relevant to emergency medicine, policing, prisons and indeed anyone working with this high-risk population. An accessible, relevant and concise guide to a challenging area of practice."

Dr Alex J. Gorton, *president Faculty of Forensic & Legal Medicine of the Royal College of Physicians*

SYMPTOMS AND SIGNS OF SUBSTANCE USE

This fourth edition of *Symptoms and Signs of Substance Use* has been thoroughly updated and revised, continuing to provide trusted information from leading experts.

There are few countries that are not touched by some aspect of substance misuse, and the consequences for individuals, families and the wider community can be devastating. This edition includes new legislation in relation to cannabis and novel psychoactive substances (NPS), as well as the following features: basic principles of treatment for the most commonly encountered substances – from tobacco and alcohol to cocaine and heroin, as well as 'designer' drugs – the legal aspects of substance use highlighted throughout, a convenient A–Z format that helps the reader find information at a glance, a bibliography that directs the reader to more authoritative information about each substance, and review questions at the end of parts I and II that help to embed learning. With specialist information clearly explained, along with a full glossary, this book is essential for all health professionals and others needing a concise and up-to-date overview of the signs and symptoms of substance use, as well as the management and treatment options available.

Those working in primary and secondary care, including general forensic medicine, emergency medicine, psychiatry, sexual offence medicine, and general practice, will find this text invaluable. This book is also an excellent resource for police officers, as well as a quick reference guide for forensic scientists, toxicologists, and postgraduate students in forensic medicine courses.

Margaret Stark is a specialist in forensic and legal medicine, consultant forensic physician, and chair of the faculty of forensic and legal medicine forensic science sub-committee.

Jason Payne-James is a specialist in forensic and legal medicine, consultant forensic physician, and lead medical examiner at Norfolk and Norwich University Hospital, Norwich, UK.

Michael Scott-Ham is a consultant forensic toxicologist with over 35 years of experience and a member of numerous professional bodies.

SYMPTOMS AND SIGNS OF SUBSTANCE USE

FOURTH EDITION

MARGARET STARK, JASON PAYNE-JAMES, AND MICHAEL SCOTT-HAM

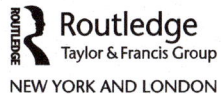

Routledge
Taylor & Francis Group

NEW YORK AND LONDON

Designed cover image: Getty Images © exdez

Fourth edition published 2025
by Routledge
605 Third Avenue, New York, NY 10158

and by Routledge
4 Park Square, Milton Park, Abingdon, Oxon, OX14 4RN

Routledge is an imprint of the Taylor & Francis Group, an informa business

First edition published by Greenwich Medical Media 1996

Third edition published by Routledge 2015

ISBN: 978-1-032-46454-1 (hbk)
ISBN: 978-1-032-46453-4 (pbk)
ISBN: 978-1-003-38173-0 (ebk)

DOI: 10.4324/9781003381730

Typeset in Galliard
by codeMantra

Thanks to the patients who taught me all about substance use and to Professor Hamid Ghodse and Dr Steven Karch who first encouraged me to develop my expertise in this area. Without Mick my partner and Amelia my daughter no writing would get done so very grateful to them for their support and encouragement.

Margaret Stark

Thanks to all my professional friends, colleagues and collaborators over the years, to the patients who have educated me, and to my supportive family.

Jason Payne-James

To the wonderful world of forensic toxicology and all of those who have assisted me during my career, and also to my wife for her support throughout.

Michael Scott-Ham

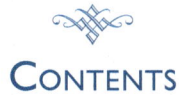

CONTENTS

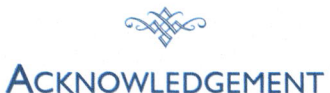

ACKNOWLEDGEMENT

Our thanks to the Taylor & Francis team, particularly Ellie Broadhurst and Pragati Sharma.

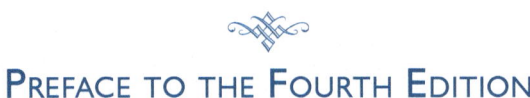

PREFACE TO THE FOURTH EDITION

Since the last edition of this book the title has been changed from *Symptoms and Signs of Substance Misuse* to *Symptoms and Signs of Substance Use*, to better reflect the aims and purpose which are to provide readers with essential information on the nature and effects of a variety of legal and non-legal substances, irrespective of the context of how they may be used.

In the decade or so since the last publication illicit drugs have become more widely available and more difficult to detect. Novel psychoactive substances have a range of effects, and for many we are as yet unaware of their particular potential for morbidity and mortality. Many are used in combination with other substances with their own range of effects. Poly-drug use results in significant complications both in terms of acute and chronic physical and mental health effects. Legal (prescribed) substances continue to be adapted for inappropriate purposes which may present with unfamiliar acute intoxication signs and symptoms, or previously undocumented effects.

Anyone who is involved with the diagnosis, treatment and management of individuals with substance use disorder needs to know the basic background of what is being used, how it is being used, and how it may present. Toxicologists and clinicians face daily challenges identifying and treating new or obscure complications of use. Legislators and law-enforcement professionals face daily challenges in determining what is legal, and how it should be regulated. This book provides information on these matters for a range of the most widely used substances and provides key information on street names, the mode of action, the potential effects and the legal status. The effects of drugs on driving are covered. The United Kingdom is used as an example for the legal status of drugs and any reader should make themselves familiar with local laws, statutes, guidance and regulation in their own jurisdiction.

Parents, families, teachers and those involved in the supervision and care of children will benefit from the information available and can use it to educate and identify issues of concern at an early stage.

With the increase in the use of substances the need for this updated resource is essential.

Margaret Stark, Jason Payne-James, Mike Scott-Ham
May 2025

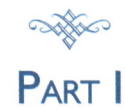

PART I

INTRODUCTION

DOI: 10.4324/9781003381730-1

Chapter 1
What Is Substance Use Disorder (SUD)?

The *Diagnostic and Statistical Manual* (DSM-5-TR™ (2023)) outlines the requirements for diagnosing SUD, which involves identifying patterns of symptoms caused by using a substance that an individual continues taking despite its negative effects. There are eleven criteria (See Table 1.1) with four categories of impaired control, physical dependence, social problems and risky use (see Table 1.2). The SUD may be further categorised by the number of symptoms present into mild (two or three), moderate (four or five), or severe (six or more).

Table 1.1 DSM-5-TR SUD

1.	Using more of a substance than intended or using it for longer than you're meant to.
2.	Trying to cut down or stop using the substance but being unable to.
3.	Experiencing intense cravings or urges to use the substance.
4.	Needing more of the substance to get the desired effect – also called tolerance.
5.	Developing withdrawal symptoms when not using the substance.
6.	Spending more time getting and using drugs and recovering from substance use.
7.	Neglecting responsibilities at home, work or school because of substance use.
8.	Continuing to use even when it causes relationship problems.
9.	Giving up important or desirable social and recreational activities due to substance use.
10.	Using substances in risky settings that put you in danger.
11.	Continuing to use despite the substance causing problems to your physical and mental health.

From: American Psychiatric Association (2023). *Diagnostic and Statistical Manual of Mental Disorders*, Fifth Edition – text revision.

DOI: 10.4324/9781003381730-2

TABLE 1.2 Categories of Symptoms

Impaired Control	Physical Dependence	Social Problems	Risky Use
Using more of a substance or more often than intended	Needing more of the substance to get the same effect (tolerance)	Neglecting responsibilities and relationships	Using in risky settings
Wanting to cut down or stop using but being unable to	Having withdrawal symptoms when a substance isn't used	Giving up activities they used to care about because of their use	Continued use despite known problems
		Inability to complete tasks at home, work or school	

From: American Psychiatric Association (2023). *Diagnostic and Statistical Manual of Mental Disorders*, Fifth Edition – text revision.

Prescription and OTC Drug Misuse

Prescription drugs and those available over-the counter (OTC) are being increasingly misused alone or in combination with illicit drugs. This may result in addictive and/or synergistic effects. There are a variety of reasons for prescription and OTC drug misuse. It may be seen as less stigmatizing and socially acceptable. Older people, adolescents, and those already on prescribed medication, including for mental illness, are more likely to misuse their prescription drugs or those available OTC. OTC drugs can be purchased legitimately from pharmacies but also from online websites and the dark web where prescription drugs can be obtained without the relevant prescription. This increases the risk of polypharmacy (the use of multiple medications) with populations with multiple morbidities, both physical and psychiatric. Some examples of the drugs misused are given in Table 1.3.

TABLE 1.3 Commonly Misused Prescribed and OTC Drugs

Prescription drugs

Benzodiazepines	alprazolam, diazepam
Bupropion	antidepressant
Gabapentinoids	gabapentin, pregabalin
Quetiapine	second generation antipsychotic
Venlafaxine	antidepressant SNRI
'Z' drugs	zolpidem, zaleplon, zopiclone

OTC

Antihistamine	chlorphenamine, diphenhydramine, promethazine
Benzydamine	NSAI
Dextromethorphan	antitussive
Hyoscine butylbromide/scopolamine	antispasmodic/antimotion sickness
Loperamide	antidiarrhoeal

Adapted from: *The Pharmaceutical Journal, PJ* November 2020, Vol 305, No 7943; 305(7943):DOI:10.1211/PJ.2020.20208538.

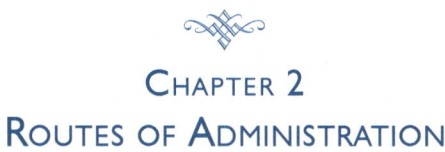

CHAPTER 2
ROUTES OF ADMINISTRATION

Routes of drug administration are the means by which a drug is taken into the body to exert its effect. The speed and amount of effect for a given dose may be modified by the different routes used for the same drug. For medical drugs there are three main routes of drug administration: topical, enteral and parenteral. Topical administration refers to when the drug is applied directly to the area where it is needed. This may be onto a skin surface or onto a cavity lining a structure (e.g. the nose and mouth). The enteral (intestinal) route of drug administration involves the drug being introduced into the intestinal (digestive) tract, which may involve taking the drug orally, infusing it, injecting it via a tube through the nose or mouth, or using suppository or enema-type applications. The third main medical route is parenteral. Parenteral administration covers the various types of injections and infusions (subcutaneous, intravenous and intramuscular).

These techniques may be used, varied or adapted by illicit drug users (both intentionally and accidentally). The main route for illicit drugs is orally – by mouth (sometimes placed under the tongue or rubbed on the gums or mouth lining or chewed) and swallowed. Taking drugs by mouth allows the drugs to pass into the stomach. Some preparations are broken down within the stomach to release drug molecules that can then pass into the intestines; this is where most absorption occurs via the intestinal walls through passive diffusion (the site varies from drug to drug) and the drug then enters the bloodstream. Drugs that are typically taken in this way are alcohol, amphetamines and some of the novel psychoactive substances (NPS), ecstasy, methadone, benzodiazepines, LSD (lysergic acid diethylamide) and magic mushrooms. Swallowing is perceived as a relatively safe way to take some drugs because the substance will be

DOI: 10.4324/9781003381730-3

slowly absorbed through the intestinal walls, resulting in effects that are less extreme and therefore less dangerous. Unfortunately, this perception may (particularly in the case of alcohol and methadone) be misleading, as this may result in a delay in the onset of severe intoxication.

The topical route is used for many drugs. Some drugs such as cocaine powder may be applied directly to the gums to achieve a very rapid effect. Direct contact with absorptive surfaces may be achieved via several methods: intranasally (or pernasally) inhaled as a pure drug into the nostrils ('sniffed', 'snorted'), by burning the drug and inhaling the fumes ('chasing', 'chasing the dragon'), or by smoking – mixing the drug with tobacco in a cigarette and inhaling the smoke.

Smoking is one of the most common routes of drug administration, and drugs that are typically smoked include tobacco, marijuana, opium, heroin, and cocaine. The smoke is drawn into the lungs and rapidly absorbed into the bloodstream. It is one of the fastest ways for someone to experience a high because the chemicals are transferred to the appropriate body receptors in seconds.

Specific side effects of long-term smoking of tobacco, or any drug, may include: a higher chance of developing heart disease, strokes and high blood pressure; mouth, throat and lung cancer; chronic obstructive pulmonary disease (including emphysema and chronic bronchitis); and bacterial pneumonia and other lung infections. An additional risk is that drugs such as cannabis and crack cocaine pose greater risks than tobacco to a smoker primarily because they need to be inhaled for a high to be experienced. A variety of everyday objects may be adapted as drug 'pipes'. Their use may not be immediately obvious. Figure 2.1 shows an asthma inhaler cover and miniature bottle of alcohol used in this way.

Vaping or vaporizing, the process of heating a substance to create a vapor, has become a recognised route of administration for a variety of drugs including synthetic cannabinoids. This may be done via commercially available vapes or e-cigarettes which can be modified for such use.

Drugs may be delivered transdermally (e.g. fentanyl and nicotine), and in the case of fentanyl there have been reports of intravenous misuse from a fentanyl patch.

The snorting of drugs (also referred to as insufflation) is conducted mostly by users of tobacco, cocaine, heroin, synthetic cathinones such as mephedrone and ketamine. Much of the snorted substance will enter the bloodstream via the mucous membrane in the nose. In general, the high is experienced within about 15 minutes of snorting. There are several

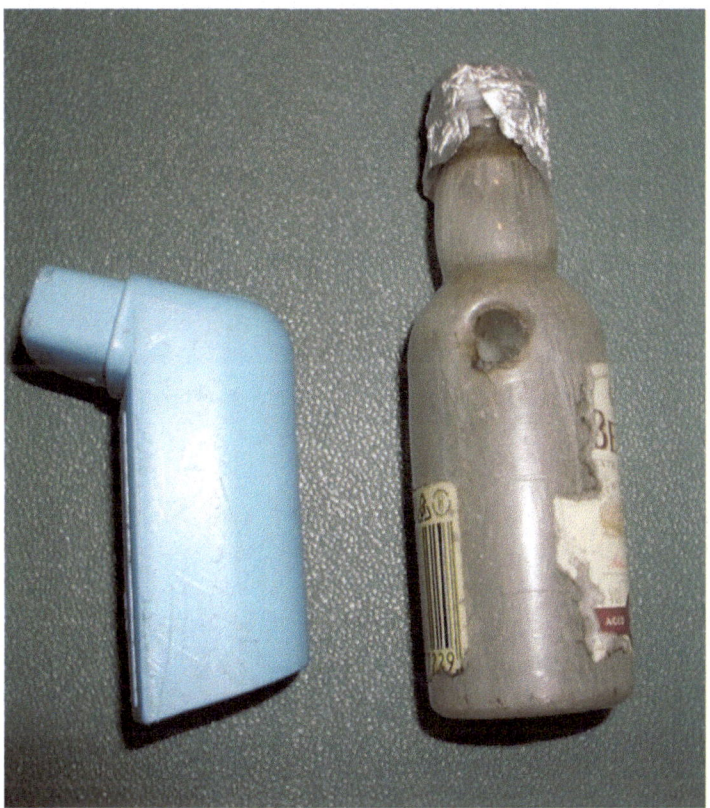

Figure 2.1 *Asthma inhaler casing and miniature bottle of whisky both used as a crack pipe*
Source: JJ Payne-James

health risks associated with this method. Probably the most widely known is that drugs such as cocaine have the potential to irreparably damage the lining of the nostrils, damage the nasal cavity, and destroy the nasal septum, the wall of cartilage between the two nostrils. This can lead to significant cosmetic disfigurement and has received wide publicity when experienced by well-known celebrities. Sharing implements (e.g., straws, bank notes) to snort drugs has the potential for transmission of infections such as hepatitis C and HIV.

A number of parenteral routes are used: intravenous ('mainlining', 'fixing') by injecting a liquid form or solution of the drug into a vein; subcutaneous ('skin-popping') by injecting into the tissue just below the skin; or intramuscular by injecting through skin and subcutaneous tissues into the muscle. Using needles is a popular method of drug administration for many opiate users because the full effects of the 'hit' are felt almost

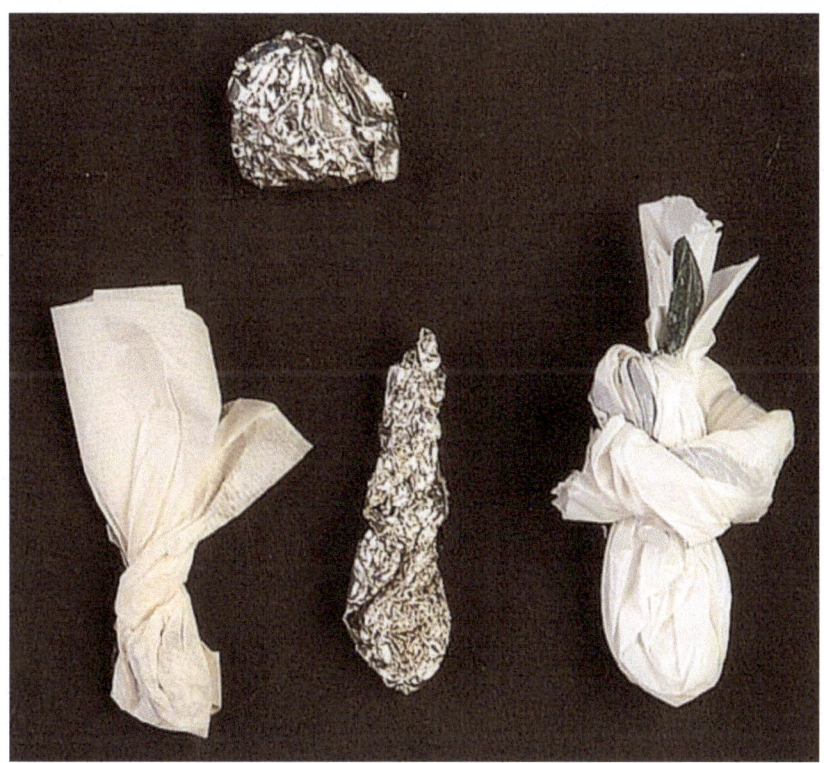

Figure 2.2 *Examples of 'wraps' of drugs (e.g. tissue and foil wraps)*
Source: JJ Payne-James

immediately, typically within a few seconds. It delivers more of the drug directly to the brain. Other drugs as crack/cocaine, amphetamine-type stimulants (ATS) and image and performance enhancing drugs (IPEDS) such as anabolic steroids may also be injected.

Injecting illicit substances is one of the more dangerous routes of administration because contaminants (of which most illicit drugs have many) that would not have entered the circulation via enteral or topical routes can enter unchallenged. This increases the risk of infection from contaminated needles or drugs, inflammation and scarring of the veins, and ulceration and vascular damage at the injection site; the latter can lead to haemorrhage, distal ischaemia, gangrene, endarteritis and thrombosis.

'Spiking' is the term generally used to describe when someone puts alcohol into a non-alcoholic drink, adds extra alcohol to an alcoholic drink or adds prescription or illegal drugs (such as benzodiazepines, or GHB, GBL) into an alcoholic or non-alcoholic drink. 'Needle spiking' is a more recent phenomenon where a drug is injected into a person without their consent. A large number of such incidents have been reported in broadcast and social media but confirmed evidence of drug administration has rarely been obtained. In recent years there appears to be an increase in spiking though it is difficult to get an accurate picture of how widespread spiking is. There are very few alleged spiking cases which are confirmed via toxicological analysis but when alleged appropriate sampling and clinical assessment are paramount. When discussing 'spiking' it is very important that the appropriate definition is used and the context understood.

In a small proportion of cases vaginal and rectal administration – insertion or placement of the drug directly into the vagina or rectum – is the route used; in these cases the drug may be absorbed rapidly across the mucosal lining.

Accidental intake occurs, for example, when drugs have been swallowed in packages, in an attempt either to conceal drugs ('swallowers') or to smuggle drugs ('stuffers', 'mules', 'body packers'), and leakage of the contents of such packages – even in small quantities – can be fatal (see Chapter 6 – Suspected Internal Drug Traffickers or SIDTs).

Drugs may present in many different ways, often as 'wraps' or 'bags' contained in paper, foil or clingfilm (Figure 2.2).

CHAPTER 3
HARM REDUCTION AND MINIMISATION

For many individuals who use drugs, the total avoidance of the drug is not an option. It is therefore unrealistic to believe that substance use will not occur. It is now recognised that, for those individuals who will continue to use drugs, it is desirable to try to reduce the amount of harm that may ensue to both the individual and the community. This approach has been termed 'harm reduction'.

Harm reduction is a term that defines policies, programs, services and actions that are intended to reduce the health, social and economic harm to individuals, communities and society associated with the use of drugs. Principles of harm reduction include provision of sterile injecting equipment, substitution therapy for opiate dependence [(OST), also referred to opioid agonist treatment (OAT) or medication-assisted treatment (MAT)], provision of vaccination, testing and treatment of infectious diseases, and drug consumption rooms providing supervised injecting facilities (see Table 3.1).

Drug-checking (testing) services provide an analysis of the content and strength of a substance and have been used at public events and venues such as music festivals. This approach remains controversial and in the UK a Home Office Licence is required. The primary aim of drug-checking services is to reduce drug-related harm. However, to accurately analyze drugs there needs to be advanced and sophisticated laboratory equipment with knowledge of the chemistry and spectral databases. If a substance is identified the risk of using such a substance may not be known. There is also a problem with interaction with other drugs, as polydrug use (the use of multiple drugs) is increasingly common.

DOI: 10.4324/9781003381730-4

Table 3.1 Principles of Harm Reduction

Provision of sterile injecting equipment:

- Needle and syringe programmes (NSP) provide sterile needles and syringes and other drug preparation equipment (cookers, filters and water for injection), in prisons and through pharmacies

Drug dependence treatment:

- Opiate substitution therapy (OST)
- Provide sterile injecting equipment in combination with OST
- Offer information, education, counselling and skills training alongside OST and needle and syringe programmes (NSPs), including in prisons

Consider vaccination:

- Hepatitis A
- Hepatitis B
- Respiratory infections such as COVID-19 and influenza
- Tetanus
- Pneumococcal
- Human papillomavirus

Testing for infectious diseases:

Routinely offer voluntary, confidential testing with informed consent for:
- HCV and HIV to all people who inject drugs
- HBV to all people who inject drugs with no/incomplete vaccination
- STIs (e.g. syphilis, chlamydia, gonorrhoea) to all people who inject drugs with STI symptoms and/or those with higher risk (e.g. multiple sexual partners, exchange of sex for money/drugs)
- TB disease to all people who inject drugs with TB signs and symptoms, and/or those with higher risk (e.g. have an exposure or predisposing underlying condition)

All people with a positive test result should be linked to care.

Infectious disease treatment:

Offer:
- Antiviral treatment for those diagnosed with HBV and eligible for treatment
- Antiviral treatment for those diagnosed with HCV
- Antiretroviral treatment for those diagnosed with HIV
- Anti-TB treatment to those with TB disease
- TB preventive treatment for people with TB infection after ruling out TB disease
- Treatment for other infectious diseases such as STIs and bacterial skin infections as clinically indicated

Ensure that there is cooperation between service providers dedicated to people who inject drugs and infectious disease care to increase linkage to care, in particular for HCV. Involvement of peer mentors may increase treatment uptake.

Drug consumption rooms providing supervised injecting facilities:

- Provide supervised injecting facilities in order to reduce injecting risk behaviour among people who inject drugs, which could as a consequence contribute to prevention of HCV and HIV transmission

Adapted from: ECDC AND EMCDDA Guidance Prevention and Control of iInfectious Diseases Among People Who Inject Drugs, November 2023 https://www.ecdc.europa.eu/en/publications-data/prevention-and-control-infectious-diseases-among-people-who-inject-drugs-2023

Harm reduction targets the causes of risks and harms. This will, in the first instance, require an understanding of what those potential harms are: (1) in a generic sense (e.g. related to modes of intake) and (2) in a drug-specific sense. The identification of specific harm, its causes and decisions about appropriate interventions require proper assessment of the problem and the actions needed. The tailoring of harm-reduction interventions to address the specific risks and harms must also take into account factors that may render people who use drugs particularly vulnerable, such as age, gender and detention.

Harm-reduction approaches should be practical, feasible, effective, safe and cost-effective. There must be an element of compassion. Stigmatisation of people who use drugs should be avoided. The use of emotive or derogatory terms such as 'drug abusers' or 'junkies' marginalises and creates barriers, and this may result in potential benefits (to the individual and society) being lost.

Common examples of harm to the individual user include contracting hepatitis or HIV infection secondary to the sharing of non-sterile needles and syringes to inject drugs. Accidental needle-stick injury from discarded injection paraphernalia creates a risk of harm to non-users. The provision of needle and syringe exchange centres in the community can reduce this risk. Hepatitis B immunisation programmes for intravenous drug users can reduce the risk of infection to the individual by reducing the incidence in the drug-using cohort, and may indirectly benefit the community by reducing costs for hospital care.

Opportunities should always be taken to educate and inform. For example a clinician may be able to provide health promotion with a brief intervention to a detainee with a SUD in police custody by means such as those shown in Table 3.2.

Naloxone and Take-home Naloxone (THN)

Naloxone is a highly effective antidote for opioids and opiates and its use is potentially lifesaving in many circumstances. It is available for injection IV and IM and as a single dose nasal spray. All HCPs should be aware of the dose and indications for administration. This should be covered in the relevant life-support training for clinicians.

THN requires training people at risk of overdose, family and friends, and service workers to administer naloxone. This is an established harm-reduction response in the UK and in many other countries.

Table 3.2 Health Promotion with Detainees in Police Custody

- Encouraging the detainee to see their general practitioner and/or attend hospital clinics to receive the appropriate care for long-term conditions
- Referring them to an on-site arrest referral/drug worker
- Providing them with information about local agencies involved in counselling and treatment of substance-related problems, such as community drug and alcohol teams, treatment centres and needle exchange schemes
- Providing them with information and advice about, and immunisation against, hepatitis B (and possibly hepatitis A)
- Checking their tetanus immunisation status if they inject drugs
- Providing advice and testing for blood-borne virus infections, hepatitis C and HIV, and referring them for treatment if required
- Educating them on the hazards of injecting drugs, particularly with regard to shared injecting equipment
- Educating them on the risks of overdose, of multiple use of substances, including alcohol, and of the variable purity of illicit drugs
- Advising them regarding the loss of tolerance and risk of fatality following reduction in regular use or a period of abstinence such as may occur following time in prison or residential rehabilitation
- Giving them contraception advice, reminders regarding cervical cancer screening, and safer sex advice and, where required, referring them to a sexual health service
- Referring them to a dentist if they have oral health problems such as dental caries, tooth erosion, or periodontal disease

From: Royal College of Psychiatrists & Faculty of Forensic and Legal Medicine (2020). *Detainees with Substance Use Disorders in Police Custody. Guidelines for Clinical Management*, Fifth Edition. College report CR 227. https://fflm.ac.uk/resources/publications/detainees-with-substance-use-disorders-in-police-custody-guidelines-for-clinical-management-5th-edition/

CHAPTER 4
DRUGS, STATUTES AND LEGAL REQUIREMENTS

This section mainly refers to legislation from the perspective of England and Wales (www.legislation.gov.uk). Those outside this jurisdiction should acquaint themselves with the relevant laws, statutes and codes relating to drugs and drug use in their locality. Drugs (both prescribed and non-prescribed) are subject to certain legal controls. Import and export of drugs controlled under the Acts are within the jurisdiction of His Majesty's Revenue and Customs.

International Conventions

The UK is obligated to follow three United Nations (UN) conventions collectively known as the Drug Control Conventions (the conventions) (see Table 4.1).

TABLE 4.1 Drug Control Conventions	
UN Single Convention on Narcotic Drugs 1961	Prohibits substances including cannabis, coca and opium-like drugs.
UN Convention of Psychotropic Substances 1971	Prohibits substances that have a psychoactive effect including psychedelics such as LSD.
UN Convention Against Illicit Traffic in Narcotic Drugs and Psychotropic Substances 1988	Provides comprehensive measures against drug trafficking, including provisions against money laundering and the diversion of precursor chemicals. It provides for international cooperation through, for example, extradition of drug traffickers, controlled deliveries and transfer of proceedings.

DOI: 10.4324/9781003381730-5

Customs and Excise Management Act 1979

Together with the Misuse of Drugs Act (see below) the Customs and Excise Management Act penalises unauthorised import or export of controlled drugs.

Misuse of Drugs Act 1971

This Act provides the legal framework for the control of drugs dividing drugs into three classes – A, B and C (examples given in Table 4.2).

TABLE 4.2	Misuse of Drugs Act 1971: Classification of drugs
Class A	Coca leaf, cocaine/crack cocaine, benzoylecgonine
	Ecstasy (MDMA), MDA, MDEA*
	Diamorphine (heroin), methadone, dipipanone, oxycodone, pethidine, fentanyl, carfentanyl
	Lysergic acid diethylamide (LSD)
	Mescaline
	Methylamphetamine, injectable amphetamines
	Psilocin
Class B	Amphetamines, methylphenidate, methylenedioxypyrovalerone MDPV
	Cannabis, cannabinol & derivatives, cannabis oil, nabiximols (oromucosalspray), cannabis resin
	Codeine, pholcodine, dihydrocodeine
	γ-Hydroxybutyrate (GHB) & γ-Butyrolactone (GBL)
	Ketamine
	Mephedrone and related cathinone derivatives
	Naphthylpyrovalerone (naphyrone)
	Phenobarbital
	Pentazocine
Class C	Anabolic steroids e.g., stanozolol, testosterone
	Benzodiazepines e.g., alprazolam, etizolam, clonazepam, chlordiazepoxide
	1-Benzylpiperazine (BZP)
	Buprenorphine
	Dextropropoxyphene
	Gabapentin & Pregabalin
	Khat
	Nitrous oxide
	Pipradol
	Tramadol
	'Z' drugs – zolpidem, zopiclone, zaleplon

* MDA, 3,4-methylenedioxyamphetamine; MDEA, 3,4-methylenedioxy-N-ethylamphetamine; MDMA, 3,4-methylenedioxy-N-methylamphetamine.

For the full list see: https://www.gov.uk/government/publications/controlled-drugs-list--2/list-of-most-commonly-encountered-drugs-currently-controlled-under-the-misuse-of-drugs-legislation.

It also states that it is an offence to:

- possess a controlled substance unlawfully
- possess a controlled substance with intent to supply it
- supply or offer to supply a controlled drug
- allow a house, flat or office to be used by people taking drugs.

The Advisory Council on the Misuse of Drugs

The Advisory Council on the Misuse of Drugs is an independent expert body, established under the Act, which advises government on drug-related issues in the UK (https://www.gov.uk/government/organisations/advisory-council-on-the-misuse-of-drugs).

Misuse of Drugs Regulations 2001

The Misuse of Drugs Regulations allows for the lawful possession and supply of controlled (illegal) drugs for legitimate purposes. They cover prescribing, administering, safe custody, dispensing, record keeping, destruction and disposal of controlled drugs to prevent diversion for misuse. Controlled drugs (CDs) are divided into five schedules (Table 4.3).

Medicines Act 1968

This Act regulates, in part, the manufacture, distribution and importation of medicinal products. Medicines are divided into three categories under the Act:

- General sales list (GSL): medicines that can be sold from any premises without supervision or advice from a doctor or pharmacist.
- Pharmacy medicines (PMs): can only be obtained from a pharmacy and are sold under the supervision of a pharmacist.
- Prescription-only medicines (POMs): must be prescribed by a doctor, a dentist or, in exceptional circumstances, another health professional.

TABLE 4.3 Misuse of Drugs Regulations: Schedule of Drugs

Schedule 1 Controlled drug (CD) licence	No recognised medical use, e.g. cannabis, LSD, mescaline. Production, possession and supply of these drugs are limited to research or other special purposes. Practitioners and pharmacists may not lawfully possess schedule 1 drugs except under licence.
Schedule 2 CD	Includes diamorphine (heroin), morphine, remifentanil, pethidine, amphetamine and cocaine. Subject to safe custody requirements requiring storage in a locked receptacle (CD cabinet). A register must be kept and comply with the regulations. The destruction of CDs in schedule 2 must be appropriately authorised and the person witnessing the destruction must be authorised to do so.
Schedule 3 CD – no register	Includes barbiturates, buprenorphine, diethylpropion, flunitrazepam, mazindol, meprobamate, midazolam, pentazocine, phentermine and temazepam. Exempt from safe custody requirements (except flunitrazepam, temazepam, buprenorphine and diethylpropion).
Schedule 4	Part 1: benzodiazepines (except temazepam, midazolam and zolpidem). Possession is an offence without a prescription. Part 2: androgenic and anabolic steroids, clenbuterol, chorionic gonadotropin, somatotrophin. No restriction on possession if part of a medicinal product.
Schedule 5	Includes preparations containing certain controlled drugs, such as codeine or pholcodine, which are exempt from full control when present in low strengths. Also nitrous oxide.

Psychoactive Substances Act 2016

A 'psychoactive substance' is defined under this Act as any substance which

a. is capable of producing a psychoactive effect in a person who consumes it, and
b. is not an exempted substance.

Exempted substances are listed in schedule 1 of the Act and cover controlled drugs, medicinal produces, alcohol, nicotine and tobacco products, caffeine and food.

This Act affects retailers who supply products that contain psychoactive substances, for example solvents and butane, but not for human consumption. The supply of these substances was previously covered by the Intoxicating Substances (Supply) Act 1985 (ISSA) which has now been repealed.

The Cigarette Lighter Refill (Safety) Regulations (1999) apply across the UK, which makes it an offence to sell butane gas lighter refills to a person under the age of 18.

Crime and Disorder Act 1988

This Act introduced enforceable drug treatment and testing orders for people convicted of crimes committed in order to maintain their drug use.

Prescribing Drugs

The law determines who can and who cannot lawfully prescribe medicines and the Royal Pharmaceutical Society Prescribing Competency Framework (2021) describes the demonstrable knowledge, skills, characteristics, qualities and behaviours for a safe and effective prescribing role (https://www.rpharms.com/resources/frameworks/prescribers-competency-framework).

The Human Medicines Regulations 2012 do not permit nurses, or other registered healthcare professionals (HCPs), who are not qualified prescribers to administer or supply prescription only medicines (POMs) unless one of three types of instruction is in place:

1. a signed prescription
2. a patient-specific direction (PSD)
3. a patient group direction (PGD).

Local arrangements can be developed to administer medicines to certain types of patients, in certain circumstances. There are different types of prescribers:

Independent prescriber: A prescribing healthcare professional who is responsible and accountable for the assessment of patients with undiagnosed or diagnosed conditions and for decisions about the clinical management required, including prescribing.

Non-medical prescriber (NMP): This term encompasses healthcare professionals (excluding doctors and dentists) working within their clinical competence as independent and/or supplementary prescribers or community practitioner nurse prescribers.

Supplementary prescribing: A voluntary partnership between a doctor or dentist and supplementary prescriber, to prescribe within an agreed patient-specific clinical management plan (CMP) with the patient's agreement. Nurses, midwives, optometrists, pharmacists, physiotherapists, podiatrists, radiographers, paramedics and dietitians may become supplementary prescribers. Once qualified, they may prescribe any medicine (including controlled drugs) within their clinical competence, according to the CMP.

Medicines can also be given by another professional with the instructions of an independent prescriber or via local arrangements.

A *patient-specific direction* (PSD) is an instruction from a doctor, dentist, or non-medical prescriber for medicines to be supplied and/ or administered to a named patient after the prescriber has assessed the patient on an individual basis.

A *patient group direction* (PGD) is a written instruction for the supply and/or administration of medicines by named healthcare professionals to groups of patients who meet the criteria specified in the PGD.

HCPs using PGDs must have been assessed as fully trained and competent to use them and must comply with the standards set by their professional regulatory body. The instruction must be agreed and signed by a senior doctor and pharmacist and authorised by an appropriate organisation. Particulars to be included in a patient group direction include the following:

- The period during which the direction is to have effect.
- The description or class of medicinal product to which the direction relates.
- The clinical situations which medicinal products of that description or class may be used to treat or manage in any form.
- Whether there are any restrictions on the quantity of medicinal product that may be sold or supplied on any one occasion and, if so, what restrictions.
- The clinical criteria under which a person is to be eligible for treatment.
- Whether any class of person is excluded from treatment under the direction and, if so, what class of person.
- Whether there are circumstances in which further advice should be sought from a doctor or dentist and, if so, what circumstances.

- The pharmaceutical form or forms in which medicinal products of that description or class are to be administered.
- The strength, or maximum strength, at which medicinal products of that description or class are to be administered.
- The applicable dosage or maximum dosage.
- The route of administration.
- The frequency of administration.
- Any minimum or maximum period of administration applicable to medicinal products of that description or class.
- Whether there are any relevant warnings to note and, if so, what warnings.
- Whether there is any follow-up action to be taken in any circumstances and, if so, what action and in what circumstances.
- Arrangements for referral for medical advice.
- Details of the records to be kept of the supply, or the administration, of products under the direction.

Doctors, registered in the UK with the General Medical Council, can prescribe controlled drugs listed in schedules 2–4, inclusive of the Misuse of Drugs Regulations 2001 under their 'professional competency' afforded to them in Regulation 7(2) of the Misuse of Drugs Regulations 2001, without the need for a Home Office licence.

However, an exception to this rule surrounds the prescription of cocaine, diamorphine and dipipanone for the treatment of addiction. These drugs can be prescribed only under a Home Office licence issued pursuant to the Misuse of Drugs (Supply to Addicts) Regulations 1997. Licences are issued to individual doctors and individual premises.

Handwriting exemptions are no longer required to exempt doctors from having to handwrite their prescriptions, although they will still have to sign and date prescriptions.

In April 2012 amendments to the Misuse of Drugs Regulations were made to allow nurse and pharmacist independent prescribers to prescribe any schedule 2–5 controlled drug within their clinical competence.

Health and Safety at Work Act 1974

The Health and Safety at Work Act 1974 places responsibilities on employers to ensure the health, safety and welfare of their employees as far as is reasonably practical as well as members of the public, and employees in turn have a responsibility to take care of their own safety and their fellow employees (https://www.hse.gov.uk/). Those self-employed also have a duty to themselves and others.

Clearly the use of drugs or alcohol by employees or knowledge by the employer of such use could mean that either or both are not fulfilling their duties under the Act.

Pre-employment screening or workplace testing programmes are becoming more common for actual conditions of employment. There are rules and regulations to ensure that any tests for drugs are carried out in a lawful and fair manner with the fully informed consent of the individual, prior to drug testing them (https://www.hse.gov.uk/alcoholdrugs/screening-testing-drugs-alcohol.htm).

The most commonly used drug test in the workplace is a urine sample as this is non-invasive, cost-effective, and can detect a broad range of drugs and their metabolites. This type of drug test is often used for pre-employment screening, post-accident testing, random testing and for cause testing when there is reasonable suspicion that an employee may be using drugs. However, increasingly saliva drug testing kits are being used.

Traffic legislation

Section 5(1)(a) of the Road Traffic Act 1988 (RTA) covering England and Wales states that a person commits an offence if a person drives or attempts to drive a motor vehicle, or is in charge of a motor vehicle on a road or other public place, when the alcohol level exceeds the limits prescribed below [section 5(1)(b)]:

- 35 micrograms (μg) alcohol in 100 millilitres (mL) of breath
- 80 milligrams per 100 mL (mg/100 mL) of blood
- 107 milligrams/100 mL urine.

Since 5 December 2014 in Scotland under the Road Traffic Act 1988 (Prescribed Limit) (Scotland) Regulations 2014 there are differing limits for alcohol compared with England and Wales:

- 22 micrograms of alcohol in 100 mL of breath
- 50 milligrams of alcohol in 100 mL of blood
- 67 milligrams of alcohol in 100 mL of urine.

Section 5A of the Road Traffic Act creates an offence of driving, attempting to drive, or being in charge of a motor vehicle on a road or public place with concentration of a specified controlled drug above specified limit (https://www.legislation.gov.uk/uksi/2014/2868/regulation/2/). The relevant drugs are listed in the Drug Driving (Specified Limits) (England and Wales) Regulations 2014 (see Table 4.4) and the Drug Driving (Specified Limits) (England and Wales) (Amendment) Regulations 2015.

There is a defence for a person charged with an offence under Section 5A if they can show that the specified controlled drug was prescribed, supplied, or purchased 'over-the-counter' (OTC) for medical or dental purposes; and that the drug was taken in accordance with advice given by the person who prescribed or supplied the drug, and in accordance with any accompanying written instructions. If police have evidence of impaired driving due to drugs, prescribed or not, then they can prosecute under the existing offence of driving whilst impaired due to drugs.

Section 4(1) of the Road Traffic Act 1988, as amended by s4 of the Road Traffic Act 1991, states that a person who, when driving or attempting to drive a mechanically propelled vehicle on a road or other public place, is unfit to drive through drink or drugs is guilty of an offence.

Section 4(2) of the Road Traffic Act 1988, as amended by s4 of the Road Traffic Act 1991, states that a person who, when in charge of a mechanically propelled vehicle which is on a road or other public place, is unfit to drive through drink or drugs is guilty of an offence.

'Drug' is defined (s11 RTA) as any intoxicant other than alcohol and so includes prescribed medications, OTC remedies and illegal substances.

A person is considered unfit to drive if that person's ability to drive is for the time being impaired [s4(5)]. For a successful prosecution, evidence is required of impairment at the time of driving and also that impairment was caused by drugs and not something else, e.g. illness or fatigue.

The Police Reform Act 2002 and the Criminal Justice (Northern Ireland) Order 2005 permit the taking of blood from incapacitated drivers for future consensual testing (section 7A RTA as amended).

The Railways and Transport Safety Act 2003 amended section 6 of the RTA to provide new powers to the police to administer preliminary tests – a preliminary breath test (section 6A), an impairment test to indicate whether a person is unfit to drive due to drink or drugs (section 6B) and a test for the presence of drugs in a person's body (section 6C).

TABLE 4.4 Specified Limits for Controlled Drugs (RTA)

Controlled drug	Limit (microgrammes per litre of blood)
Benzoylecgonine	50
Clonazepam	50
Cocaine	10
Delta-9-Tetrahydrocannabinol	2
Diazepam	550
Flunitrazepam	300
Ketamine	20
Lorazepam	100
Lysergic Acid Diethylamide	1
Methadone	500
Methylamphetamine	10
Methylenedioxymethamphetamine	10
6-Monoacetylmorphine	5
Morphine	80
Oxazepam	300
Temazepam	1000

Transport and Works Act 1992

Section 27(1) of the Transport and Works Act 1992 states that it is an offence for any of the following people to carry out their work while unfit through drink or drugs; namely a train or tram driver, guard, conductor or signalman, or anybody who works on a transport system in which they can control or affect the movement of a vehicle or works in a maintenance capacity or as a supervisor or lookout for people working in a maintenance capacity.

Under section 27(2) of the Act it is an offence for these people to carry out their work after having consumed more alcohol than the prescribed limit.

Drugs Act 2005

The Drugs Act 2005 amended the Police and Criminal Evidence Act and the Misuse of Drugs Act 1971 to increase the powers of police and the court in relation to drug control. Police are allowed to test drug offenders on arrest (as opposed to on charging), requiring those testing positive to undergo treatment. It also empowers police to authorise intimate searches, X-rays and ultrasound scans on people suspected of having concealed class A drugs with the intention to supply or export them.

CHAPTER 5
THE MEDICAL AND HEALTH COMPLICATIONS OF SUBSTANCE USE

Substance use disorder (SUD) can result in medical and other health complications that may be specific to the particular substance of use (see Part II, Specific Drugs) or generic – in that the complications are caused by the mode of substance use. Such complications may be the first indicator of a substance use problem in the absence of acute or chronic symptoms and signs of specific drugs.

Acute intoxication with a drug can lead to minor side effects such as vomiting, confusion, drowsiness and fainting, or more serious effects such as seizures, unconsciousness, sepsis and death. With chronic usage additional physical and psychological health effects may occur.

Drug-related deaths in the UK have been increasing in recent years and almost half of all drug-poisoning deaths continue to involve an opiate. Cocaine deaths are on the rise as are deaths from polydrug use, for example the use of benzodiazepines and gabapentinoids are increasingly seen with the use of heroin and other opiates increasing the risk of overdose.

Overdoses related to opioid use are mainly characterised by respiratory depression, whereas those due to cocaine are characterised by cardiac-related events such as myocardial infarction or stroke, and ecstasy by hyperthermia or hyponatraemia.

Any patient who is known to use or suspected of using substances including alcohol should have a full history and clinical examination at regular intervals to determine the risks or establish the presence of any treatable or new complication. This should be done with the consent of the individual. A comprehensive history should be obtained regarding past and present substance use (Table 5.1). In relation to alcohol the

DOI: 10.4324/9781003381730-6

TABLE 5.1 Information to be Sought When Assessing Past and Present Drug Use

Type(s) of substance(s) used
Form of substance used (e.g. cannabis resin, skunk, weed)
How long each substance has been used
How often each substance has been used – daily vs occasional (recreational usage)
Quantity of each drug taken per day (average day)
Amount spent on drug per day (average day)
Method of administration (noting sites of any injection if used)
The time of the last dose(s) of substances
The amount used in the past 24–48 hours
Prescribed medication, especially opiate substitution treatment (OST)
Use of alcohol (brief MAST, CAGE and AUDIT questionnaires may be useful in the assessment)
Use of tobacco
Use of over-the-counter (OTC) medicines

following assessment questionnaires may be useful: Brief MAST, CAGE and AUDIT (see Appendix D).

The physical examination should also establish whether there is clinical evidence the individual is intoxicated or withdrawing (using the Clinical Opiate Withdrawal Scale in Appendix C (COWS) and Clinical Institute Withdrawal Assessment of Alcohol Scale, Revised (CIWA-Ar), in Appendix B as appropriate) from alcohol and /or a drug(s) at that time and identify relevant medical conditions. The physical examination should include an external physical examination of the body looking for needle marks and needle tracks in people who inject drugs (PWID). Table 5.2 shows key features that may need to be assessed.

If there is clear evidence of current intoxication, it is appropriate to document baseline consciousness level, using ACVPU (alert, confusion (new), voice, pain, unresponsive) or the Glasgow Coma Scale (GCS https://www.glasgowcomascale.org/), although it is important to be aware that the GCS scale is specifically for head injury and not validated for those under the influence of drugs or alcohol (Table 5.3) and other vital signs such as pulse, blood pressure, temperature, oxygen saturation, blood glucose and respiratory rate. A brief mental state examination should also be performed. The remainder and extent of the physical examination will be determined on a case-by-case basis. However, if faced with an acutely unwell patient the use of the National Early Warning Score (NEWS2) is recommended to help standardise the assessment

TABLE 5.2 Examination

Physical examination

The following baseline assessments are essential for all examinations of those suspected of using alcohol and/or drugs

- Conscious level (ACVPU and/or GCS)
- Blood pressure
- Pulse rate
- Temperature
- Respiratory rate
- Blood glucose
- Oxygen saturation
- Eye examination: pupil size (Figure 5.1)
  - o Reaction to light
  - o Eye movements (nystagmus)
  - o Convergence
  - o Conjunctival appearance

Other observations

- Skin colour – pallor/flushed
- Speech – content/articulation
- Presence of needle tracks, other skin stigmata
- Presence of tremor
- Yawning, lacrimation, rhinorrhoea
- Gooseflesh, sweating
- Bowel sounds
- Coordination, Romberg's (balance) test
- Assessment of gait
- Auscultation of the heart and lungs
- COWS and/or CIWA-Ar scores

Brief mental state examination

- Appearance (clothing)
- Behaviour
- Speech (rate and volume)
- Thought disorder (delusions)
- Disordered perceptions (hallucinations, illusions)
- Obsessive–compulsive behaviours
- Mood (euphoric, withdrawn, depressed)
- Biological symptoms (loss of appetite, disturbed sleep pattern)
- Cognitive function (orientation in time place and person, memory, concentration)
- Risk behaviours: harm to self and others

and response to acute illness with an aggregate score covering respiration rate, oxygen saturation, systolic blood pressure, pulse rate, level of consciousness or new confusion, and temperature (https://www.rcp.ac.uk/improving-care/resources/national-early-warning-score-news-2/).

TABLE 5.3 Glasgow Coma Scale

EYE OPENING

Criterion	Observed	Rating	Score
Open before stimulus		Spontaneous	4
After spoken or shouted request		To sound	3
After fingertip stimulus		To pressure	2
No opening at any time, no interfering factor		None	1
Closed by local factor		Non testable	NT

VERBAL RESPONSE

Criterion	Observed	Rating	Score
Correctly gives name, place and date		Orientated	5
Not orientated but communication coherently		Confused	4
Intelligible single words		Words	3
Only moans/groans		Sounds	2
No audible response, no interfering factor		None	1
Factor interfering with communication		Not testable	NT

BEST MOTOR RESPONSE

Criterion	Observed	Rating	Score
Obeys two-part request		Obeys commands	6
Brings hand above clavicle to stimulus on head neck		Localising	5
Bends arm at elbow rapidly but features not predominantly abnormal		Normal flexion	4
Bends arm at elbow, features clearly predominantly abnormal		Abnormal flexion	3
Extends arm at elbow		Extension	2
No movement in arms/legs, no interfering factor		None	1
Paralysed or other limiting factor		Not testable	NT

Habitual smokers of certain drugs develop chronic wheeze, which may be improved by abstinence from the drug or use of bronchodilators. Most individuals who have smoked or chased heroin or crack cocaine will have intermittent wheeze (which may be particularly evident during opiate withdrawal).

Many drugs can be injected and people who inject drugs (PWIDs) are vulnerable to a wide range of viral and bacterial infections. Many of the injection-related complications, irrespective of the drug injected, are caused by either sharing (although this has decreased in recent years), or repeated use of non-sterile needles.

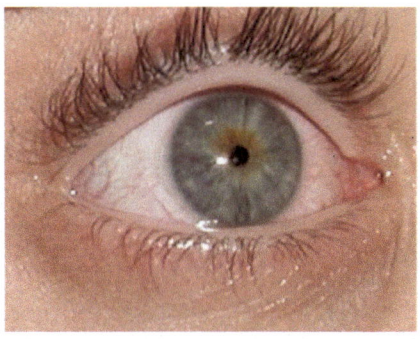 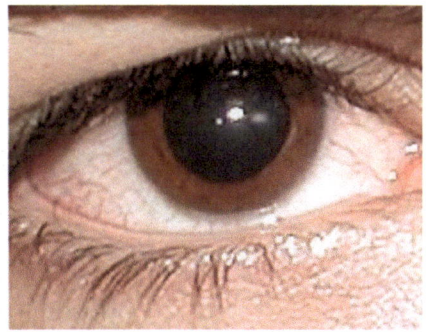

Figure 5.1   *(a) Pin-point pupil caused by acute intoxication with heroin. (b) Dilated pupil caused by intoxication with MDMA (as stimulant).*
Source: JJ Payne-James.

HCV is the most common BBV infection among PWID in the UK increasing from 47% in 2012 to 57% in 2021. HIV prevalence remains low and stable; 1.5% of PWID surveyed in 2021 were living with HIV in England, Wales and NI (EWNI). In the UK hepatitis B virus infection among PWIDs has declined with 5.9% in 2021, probably due to the increase in hepatitis B immunisation. However, the vaccine provision to PWID was substantially reduced during the COVID-19 pandemic.

Adulterants may be defined as any substance or organism found in illicit drugs at the point of purchase other than the active ingredient. The presence of adulterants can increase the risk of morbidity and mortality.

PWIDs often have abscesses, sores or open wounds, which may be infected with *Staphylococcus aureus*, group A streptococci and methicillin-resistant and methicillin-sensitive *Staphylococcus aureus* (MRSA). Cases of botulism and tetanus have occurred in PWIDs. In the UK 2021, there were two cases of wound botulism in PWID and one case of tetanus with a history of recent drug injection but no cases of anthrax.

Table 5.4 lists the most common medical complications of substance use and some of the rarer conditions that should be looked for at an acute assessment.

There are high rates of co-occurrence of mental disorder and substance use disorder. A brief mental state examination should be performed in all suspected cases, considering the appearance, behaviour, speech, presence of thought, perceptual and/or obsessive–compulsive

TABLE 5.4 Examples of Potential Complications of Substance Use

Vascular

May be short term or longer term:

- Accidental intra-arterial (as opposed to intravenous) injection may cause vascular spasm with ischaemia
- False aneurysm
- Thrombophlebitis
- Thrombosis
- Embolus
- Vascular spasm

Vascular spasm, thrombosis and embolus if severe and untreated can result in gangrene and loss of digits or limbs.

Intravenous injection may be followed by:

- Localised superficial thrombophlebitis
- Deep vein thrombosis
- Pulmonary embolism

Chronic complications include:

- Limb swelling (a mixture of lymphoedema and post-phlebitic changes) (Figure 5.2a)
- Varicose eczema
- Varicose ulcers (Figure 5.2b)

Infective complications of injection

Short-term complications:

- Abscess (Figure 5.3)
- Bacteraemia/septicaemia
- Cellulitis (local – chemical and infective)
- Thrombophlebitis

Longer-term complications:

- Endocarditis (always look for splinter haemorrhages, anaemia)
- Hepatitis:

    o A (several large outbreaks have occurred in PWID)
    o B (2021 5.9% of PWID)
    o C (2021 57% of intravenous drug users)
    o Chronic hepatitis: cirrhosis may result and primary hepatocellular carcinoma
    o Hepatitis D virus infection may be superimposed on hepatitis B virus infection

- Human immunodeficiency virus (HIV) (2021) UK 1.5% of PWID
- Necrotising fasciitis
- Osteomyelitis (haematogenous)

- Respiratory:
  - o lung abscess
  - o tuberculosis (associated with homelessness, HIV, malnutrition and immunological suppression)
  - o septic arthritis

- Non-infective complications
  - o Anaphylaxis
  - o Constipation (chronic opiate use)
  - o Dental decay (especially with methadone use, cocaine and methamphetamine users)
  - o Local ulceration (at injection site) (Figure 5.4)
  - o Malnutrition
  - o Overdose (accidental)
  - o Pneumothorax (after forced inhalation of drugs such as cocaine)
  - o Pulmonary infarction
  - o Respiratory wheeze (non-infective – worse on withdrawal from opiates)

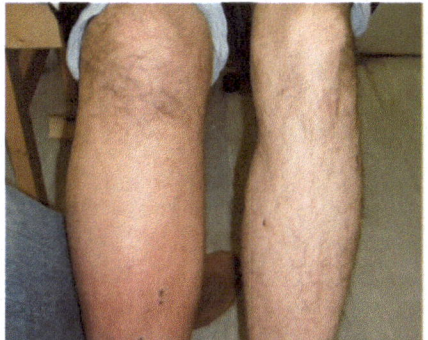 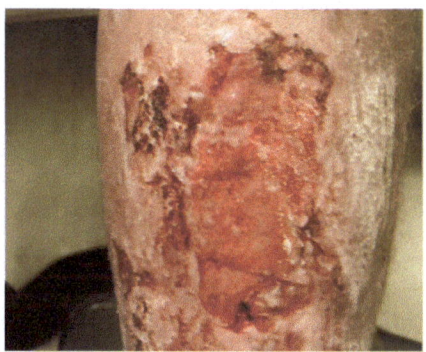

Figure 5.2 *(a) Right-sided post-phlebitic limb secondary to repeated injection to right femoral vein. (b) Venous ulcer secondary to repeated deep venous thrombosis caused by injection to femoral vein.*
Source: JJ Payne-James

disorders, mood, biological symptoms, cognitive function and risk behaviours (see Table 5.2).

Such an assessment of an acutely disturbed patient should differentiate whether the patient has one of the following: a panic reaction; an organic mental state characterised by disorientation in time and space; impaired mental functioning, often with perceptual disturbances such as hallucinations or illusions; or a psychotic illness characterised by delusions and hallucinations in a setting of clear consciousness, often with evidence of thought disorder and lack of insight.

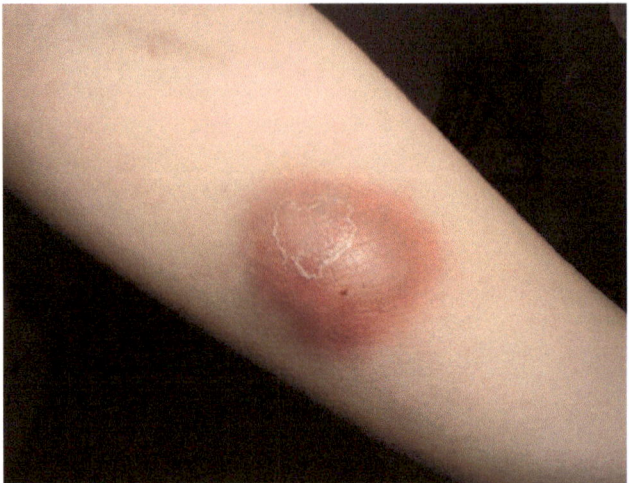

Figure 5.3 *Fluctuant abscess to forearm caused by intravenous drug injection (note gooseflesh caused by associated opiate withdrawal)*
Source: JJ Payne-James

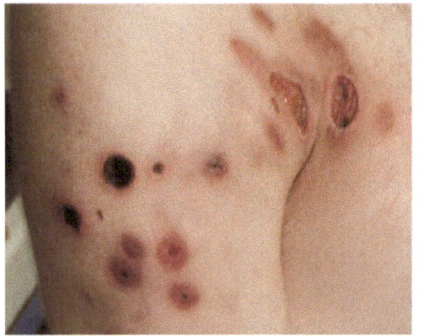 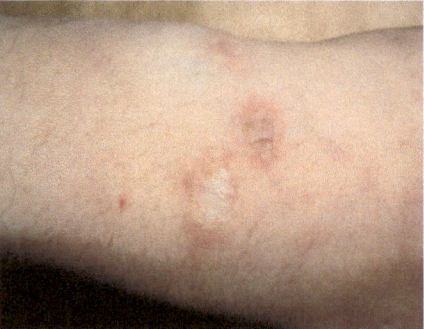

Figure 5.4 *(a) Skin ulceration caused by repeated drug injection. (b) Mature scars caused by repeated drug injection.*
Source: ©JJ Payne-James

Chronic substance use disorder is also associated with psychiatric disorders such as schizophrenia and personality disorders. Depression, bipolar disorder and anxiety disorders, including generalised anxiety, panic and post-traumatic stress disorder (PTSD), are associated with an increased lifetime risk of substance abuse. Traumatic events, such as childhood sexual abuse, may increase an individual's vulnerability and increase the likelihood of use of psychoactive substances. People who use substances have higher rates of completed and attempted suicide compared with the general population.

Older people

In the past decade there has been an increase in the number of people with SUD in drug treatment in the community maintained on opioid substitution treatment (OST), often with complex co-morbidities, prescribed multiple medicines. These have been described as 'early-onset users' and are different to a sometimes quite distinct population of 'late-onset users' of substances who may have begun using them regularly only later in life, often following stressful life events or lifestyle changes (for example retirement, marital breakdown, social isolation, increasing morbidity or bereavement.

Psychiatric comorbidities are particularly common in older people, including intoxication and delirium, withdrawal syndromes, anxiety, depression and cognitive changes with or without dementia. High rates of mental illness and cognitive disorders result in complex comorbidity in this group, with older people, for example, using alcohol with prescribed and over-the-counter (OTC) medication.

Toxidromes

A toxidrome describes a syndrome of symptoms and signs caused by a dangerous (toxic) level of toxins/drugs/substances in the blood.

Sympathomimetic Toxidrome

Sympathomimetic toxidrome results from misuse of stimulant drugs such as ecstasy, cocaine methamphetamine, amphetamine, and ATS. Clinical features are outlined in Table 5.5.

TABLE 5.5 Sympathomimetic Toxidrome

Altered mental state, euphoria, agitation, delirium, hallucinations
Increased pulse, blood pressure, temperature (hyperpyrexia)
Dysrhythmias
Dilated pupils (mydriasis)
Seizures

Opiates

Intoxication and overdose with opioids such as heroin, morphine, methadone, and oxycodone is increasingly common with increasing mortality. Clinical features are outlined in Table 5.6.

Serotonin Syndrome

Serotonin syndrome results from an excess of serotonin in the central nervous system (CNS) and usually develops over a period of 24 hours. It is characterised by hyperpyrexia associated with secondary complications, including rhabdomyolysis (breakdown of skeletal muscle), disseminated intravascular coagulation and acute kidney injury. These toxic effects are more likely with the co-administration of certain drugs, for example the use of ecstasy with prescribed drugs such as antidepressants, in particular selective serotonin reuptake inhibitors (SSRIs), e.g. fluoxetine, selective serotonin/noradrenaline reuptake inhibitors (SNRIs), e.g. venlafaxine, or monoamine oxidase inhibitors (MAOIs) such as moclobemide. Signs and symptoms of serotonin syndrome are outlined in Table 5.7.

TABLE 5.6 Opioid Toxidrome

Decreased pulse, blood pressure, temperature (hyperpyrexia)
Pin-point pupils (miosis)
Respiratory depression
CNS depression, coma
Pulmonary oedema

TABLE 5.7 Serotonin Syndrome

Agitation
Diarrhoea
Heavy sweating not associated with physical activity
Fever
Mental status changes such as confusion or hypomania
Muscle spasms (myoclonus)
Overactive reflexes (hyperreflexia)
Shivering
Tremor
Uncoordinated movements (ataxia)

Neuroleptic malignant syndrome (NMS)

NMS is a rare, but life-threatening, idiosyncratic reaction to neuroleptic medications, such as antipsychotics. Individuals may present with altered mental status, fever, muscular rigidity and autonomic dysfunction. The development of NMS takes days or weeks.

Anticholinergic Toxidrome

Anticholinergic syndrome may result from misuse of drugs such as tricyclic antidepressants (TCADs), antihistamines, antipsychotics and antiparkinsonian. Clinical features of the syndrome are outlined in Table 5.8.

TABLE 5.8 Anticholinergic Toxidrome

Agitation, altered mental state
Dry mouth (mucous membranes)
Hot flushed skin
Constipation
Urinary retention
Bowel obstruction decreased bowel sounds
Blurred vision
Dilated pupils
Increased pulse, respiratory rate and blood pressure
Hyperthermia

TABLE 5.9 Clinical Features of Alcohol, Sedative, Hypnotic Toxidrome (not all have to be present)

Alteration in mental state, labile effect
Sedation
Concentration/attention/memory difficulties
Slurred speech
Increased pulse, blood pressure
Skin flushing
Nystagmus
Pupil size – may be normal or dilated
Sluggish pupillary reaction to light
Poor coordination
Romberg's positive Intoxication/Overdose
Respiratory depression
Central nervous system depression, coma
Depressed or absent corneal, gag or deep tendon reflexes
Cardiovascular system depression

Alcohol, Sedative, Hypnotic Toxidrome

Alcohol, benzodiazepines and barbiturates produce a similar toxidrome (see Table 5.9).

Acute Behavioural Disturbance

Acute behavioural disturbance (ABD) is an overarching term for the clinical presentation of several conditions, see Table 5.10. The commonest causes in forensic practice are related to the use of drugs and mental health conditions.

Cases of suspected ABD must be taken directly to the emergency department (ED) of the local hospital especially if the detainee exhibits any of the following signs: tactile hyperthermia (hot to touch), constant or near constant physical activity, extreme agitation/aggression (Figure 5.5).

The most significant clinical features include tactile hyperthermia ('hot to touch'), does not fatigue, naked/inappropriately clothed, rapid breathing, sweating profusely, disproportionate strength, pain tolerance, constant/near constant activity, glass attraction-destruction, and not responsive to others' presence (e.g. law enforcement personnel).

TABLE 5.10 The Differential Diagnosis of ABD

Akathisia
Anticholinergic syndrome (e.g. antihistamines)
CNS infection (meningitis/encephalitis)
Heat exhaustion
Head injury
Hypoglycaemia
Hypoxia
Neuroleptic malignant syndrome
Psychiatric disorders
Sedative (e.g. alcohol, benzodiazepine, GHB and related drugs, rarely, opioid) withdrawal
Seizures
Sepsis
Serotonin syndrome
Stimulant or synthetic cannabinoid receptor agonist (SCRA) intoxication
Thyroid storm

From: *Acute Behavioural Disturbance* (2024). Faculty of Forensic and Legal Medicine (FFLM).

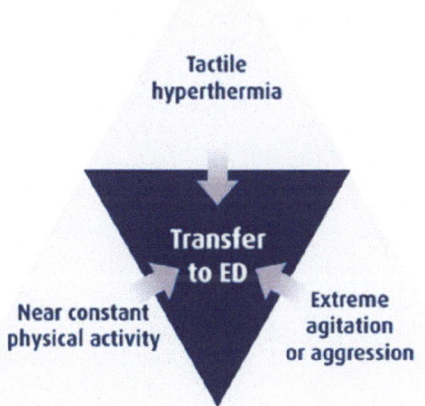

Figure 5.5 *Signs of suspected cases of ABD.*
Source: Acute Behavioural Disturbance (2024). FFLM.

The management of an individual who is suspected of having ABD needs a collaborative approach, between police, paramedics, and the emergency department, with early recognition, intervention, and proactive treatment. De-escalation should always be tried. Treatment in the pre-hospital environment may need to be considered to transfer the individual to hospital and prevent deterioration of the clinical condition.

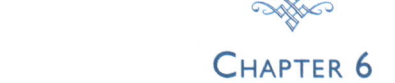

Chapter 6
Suspected Internal Drug Traffickers

Individuals who swallow drugs to avoid detection by authorities are referred to by a number of names, including 'drug stuffers' or 'contact precipitated concealers'. Drug swallowers tend to ingest small amounts of drugs, e.g. ecstasy, cannabis or cocaine, with low levels of purity often inadequately wrapped in clingfilm. Such behaviour is not uncommon and may be associated with harmful effects. Police policy has been to treat such detainees as a medical emergency and transfer them immediately to hospital for assessment. Individuals may also place drugs in their vagina and/or rectum, so-called 'body pushers'.

Appropriate training for healthcare professionals and authorities such as police, prison or security staff is essential. There must be a heightened awareness of the possibility of drug ingestion because individuals who are detained by the relevant authorities are unlikely to disclose that they have swallowed illicit substances. At any stage after ingestion a medical emergency may occur, caused by the rupture of a drug package. Signs of intoxication may occur within 6 hours but may be delayed until the packaging has been destroyed and this may take up to 24 hours. Sudden death is a risk from massive overdose of the ingested drug, e.g. cocaine. The risk of harm may also depend on whether the individual is a naïve user or a habituated, with some tolerance to the effects of the drug concealed, e.g. opioids. Details of the packaging should always be obtained in any assessment of detainees who have swallowed drugs.

Body packers or 'mules' are individuals who deliberately ingest packages of drugs such as cocaine, amphetamine-type stimulants (ATSs) and heroin, often in large quantities, to avoid detection by the authorities. The drugs are maybe of high purity and packaged using machine-manufactured material that does not leak. The packages may be swallowed

DOI: 10.4324/9781003381730-7

with anticholinergic drugs to reduce intestinal motility and prevent the passage of the drugs before the end of the proposed journey.

In England and Wales police have powers to authorise intimate searches, X-rays and ultrasound scans on people suspected of having concealed class A drugs with the intent to supply and export them. However low dose CT scan (LDCT) of the abdomen/pelvis is the investigation of choice for suspected internal drug traffickers (SIDTs). Any such test may be performed only with the consent of the individual. If acute symptoms and signs develop, due to obstruction, ileus, worsening toxicity, then urgent CT with referral to the surgeons will be required.

Healthcare professionals may be asked to perform intimate searches for drugs and should attend to assess the person arrested but only proceed to an intimate search with the person's fully informed consent.

It should be remembered that urinary and/or blood toxicology screens should not be used to guide the management of when a SIDT is fit for discharge as this may be negative due to good packaging.

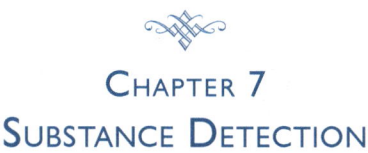

CHAPTER 7
SUBSTANCE DETECTION

There are many different kinds of healthcare professionals that may need to test individuals for drugs to help control substance use, including occupational health teams, general practitioners, drug clinics and, increasingly, employers. Such testing requires consideration, including a range of ethical, moral and statutory issues.

Testing may be required for the police investigations of drug-facilitated crime (DFC) including drugs and driving, sexual assault (including 'date-rape', more properly referred to as drug-facilitated sexual assault – DFSA), murders, suspicious deaths, and poisonings. A coroner (in England & Wales), when carrying out a death investigation, may need to know whether an individual has died through ingestion of a drug, or whether a drug played any other role in the death. Family courts may be interested in drug use by parties in care proceedings. Prior drug use by parties involved in insurance claims, e.g. motor vehicle crashes, may be relevant.

Accreditation requirements for laboratories undertaking toxicological work varies by country but also often by the type of work being undertaken. Some work arenas are highly regulated whereas others have no regulatory or accreditation requirements. Accreditation adds to analytical costs.

One of the most important factors to consider is to ensure that the medium being tested, and the analytical technique used, is fit for purpose. All drugs will be metabolised to some extent and it is essential to test for the correct compound, e.g. there is little point in analysing for a parent drug when it is very quickly, or completely, metabolised.

Different techniques have different limits of detection (the lowest concentration of drug that is reliably detectable), and it can be misleading, if not potentially dangerous, to use an inappropriate technique that does not have sufficient sensitivity to detect the compound of interest.

DOI: 10.4324/9781003381730-8

Required limits of detection for compounds in a workplace drug-testing (WDT) scenario are much higher than are required in forensic casework and to use WDT methods, with their associated sensitivities, for forensic detection would result in significant findings being missed in many cases.

It is also important to consider the difference between qualitative and quantitative/confirmatory analytical methods. The former are generally used to screen samples for the presence or absence of compounds, often drug groups that are chemically similar, but a positive result is not conclusive proof of the presence of an analyte. The latter are used to confirm the presence of the compound and measure the amount present, when required. There will be differences between laboratories in methods employed, limits of detection and the amount of information supplied in the analytical report/certificate, all of which need to be taken into consideration when assessing the result.

Screening methods frequently employ immunoassay techniques although, increasingly, high pressure liquid chromatography (HPLC), coupled with mass spectrometry, is used for screening (LC-MS). The latter method may be targeted, i.e. screening for a list of named compounds, or a so-called general unknown screening can be used in which all compounds detectable by the method will be looked for. In recent years it has become increasingly challenging to be able to detect and identify drugs with the widespread availability of many new designer drugs, commonly known as novel psychoactive substances (NPS), most of which have been synthesised illicitly and for which no certified reference materials (CRMs) are available to use as standards during analysis. In this ever-changing and expanding marketplace, new drugs are being encountered frequently. If there is a requirement to detect all of these compounds, accurate mass LC-MS is an analytical must.

Quantitative and confirmatory techniques almost all employ mass spectrometry, often with gas chromatographic separation but, increasingly, with HPLC separation. Although many NPS may be detected using accurate mass screening methods, it is not possible to accurately measure the concentration present in a biological fluid, without a CRM. Although many compounds will have a specific accurate mass, and therefore potentially be identifiable, the situation is confused by an increasing number of compounds being chemically very similar to others, some merely being positional isomers of another compound, thereby sharing the same molecular formula. Consequently, such compounds may not be separable from others using certain MS techniques. Some techniques permit retrospective data processing to enable searches for new drugs to be performed. Care should thus be taken in interpreting results.

Samples available for analysis include urine, blood, hair and oral fluid. Blood may offer a window of detection of up to 72 hours for some drugs, with urine offering a longer window of up to occasionally 5 days, but both being dependent on the pharmacokinetics of the drug in question. Some drugs are only detectable for much shorter periods of time in both blood and urine. Typical timeframes for drug detection are 24 hours in blood and 48 hours in urine. Oral fluid detection times are generally shorter, up to 24 hours, whereas hair may offer a very much longer window of detection, measured in months or even years if the hair length is sufficient. Hair can be taken 6 weeks after the index event.

In some situations, blood offers the advantage of possibly providing an interpretation in answer to questions such as how much drug has been taken and when, whereas urine is less open to interpretation. Oral fluid potentially offers an interpretation similar to blood but paucity of data currently precludes detailed interpretation for most drugs.

Hair analysis may offer some limited interpretation if carried out in an appropriate manner; e.g. if analysed segmentally, it may be possible to give an indication of whether a drug has been taken chronically or acutely, which may be relevant in forensic casework, but also in assessing possible drug tolerance in other situations. If no segmental analysis is performed, the only question that can be answered is whether the drug has been taken, assuming that the sensitivity of the method used was appropriate.

Clinicians should be aware of the local recommendations, including timescales, for taking forensic specimens (https://fflm.ac.uk/resources/publications/recommended-equipment-for-obtaining-forensic-samples-from-complainants-and-suspects/) and have access to appropriate forensic kits, validated and quality-controlled for toxicology specimen of blood, hair and urine (https://fflm.ac.uk/about/board-and-committees/forensic-science-subcommittee/).

Chain-of-custody procedures and measures to prevent sample contamination should be followed in all instances; failure to do so may result in the analyses not being admissible as evidence.

TABLE 7.1 Characteristics of some common drugs

Drug	Half-life (h)[a]	Typical Blood Concentration (mg/L)	Major Metabolites (pharmacologically active or inactive)
Amphetamine	7–34 (urine pH dependent)	0.02–0.20	Benzoic acid, hippuric acid (both inactive)
Cannabis (THC)	Highly variable – THC[b] rapidly disappears from bloodstream and is deposited in body fat from where it leaches out at a rate dependent on frequency of use	0.001–0.010 (THC) 0.001–0.050 (carboxy-THC)	Hydroxy-THC (active) Carboxy-THC (inactive)
Cocaine	0.7–1.5	0.05–0.30 (cocaine)	Benzoylecgonine, methylecgonine, ecgonine (all inactive)
Benzoylecgonine (cocaine metabolite)	5–8	0.1–1.0 (benzoylecgonine)	
Diamorphine (heroin)	0.03–0.10 (diamorphine) 0.10–0.40 (6-MAM) 2–3 (morphine)	Diamorphine ND[c] 0.01–0.10 (6-MAM) 0.01–0.10 (morphine) 0.10–0.50 (morphine-3-glucuronide)	6-Monoacetylmorphine (6-MAM), morphine (both active), morphine-3-glucuronide (inactive), morphine-6-glucuronide (active)
Methadone	15–55	0.03–0.30	EDDP,[d] EMDP[e] (both inactive)
Diazepam	21–37	0.05–2.00 (diazepam)	Desmethyldiazepam, temazepam, oxazepam (all active)
Desmethyldiazepam	40–99	0.10–3.00 (desmethyldiazepam)	
Diazepam metabolite)			
Ketamine	2–4	0.20–1.00 (ketamine) 0.05–0.10 (norketamine)	Norketamine (active)
Methamphetamine	6–15 (urine pH dependent)	0.02–0.30	Amphetamine (active), parahydroxymethamphetamine
Methylenedioxy-methamphetamine (MDMA)	4–8	0.10–0.35	Methylenedioxyamphetamine (MDA, active)
γ-Hydroxybutyrate (GHB)	0.30–1.00	80–250	Succinic acid (inactive)

a Half-life – $t_{\frac{1}{2}}$: the time taken for a concentration of a drug to decrease to half of the peak concentration.

b THC: tetrahydrocannabinol.

c ND: not detected.

d EDDP: 2-ethylidene-1,5-dimethyl-3,3-diphenylpyrrolidine

e EMDP: is 2-ethyl-5-methyl-3,3-diphenylpyrrolidine;.

CHAPTER 8
PART I SELF-ASSESSMENT QUESTIONS

1. How would you diagnose the severity of SUD?
2. What is 'spiking'? What drugs are commonly used?
3. Outline the five principles of harm reduction.
4. What is the legal status of nitrous oxide in the UK?
5. How are novel psychoactive substances (NPS) controlled in the UK?
6. What physical signs might lead you to suspect someone had used a stimulant drug?
7. Outline the clinical presentation of an overdose with etizolam.
8. What is Serotonin Syndrome? Provide three examples of drugs that may cause this syndrome.
9. Outline the vascular complications that may occur when people inject drugs.
10. What are the three signs in cases of suspected ABD that indicate the individual should be taken directly to the emergency department (ED) of the nearest hospital?
11. What is the difference between 'drug swallowers' and 'drug packers'?
12. What are the recommended timescales to take forensic specimens for blood, urine and hair?

DOI: 10.4324/9781003381730-9

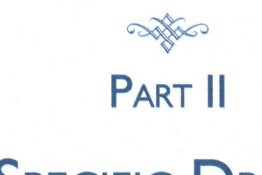

PART II

SPECIFIC DRUGS

A
Alcohol
Aminoindanes, indoles and benzofurans
Amphetamine-type Stimulants

B
Barbiturates
Benzodiazepines

C
Cannabis
Cocaine

E
Ecstasy

G
Gabapentinoids

H
γ-Hydroxybutyrate and Related Compounds

K
Ketamine
Khat

DOI: 10.4324/9781003381730-10

L

LSD

N

Nitrites

Nitrous Oxide

O

Opiates/Opioids

P

Phencyclidine

Phenethylamines

Piperazines

Pipradrols

S

Synthetic Cannabinoids

Synthetic Cathinones

T

Tobacco

Tryptamines

V

Volatile Substances

Z

'Z' Drugs

Self-Assessment Questions

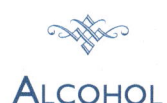

Alcohol

Principal Drugs

Ethanol (ethyl alcohol), methanol (methyl alcohol, wood alcohol, wood spirits). Ethanol and methanol are formulated together as methylated spirits (meths).

Common Street Names

Booze, hooch, tipple, meths, firewater, hard stuff, liquid courage, sauce.

Mechanism of Action

Ethanol is a central nervous system (CNS) depressant; producing pharmacological effects by enhancing λ-aminobutyric acid (GABA) transmission; consequently abrupt cessation of the drugs will result in a reduction in GABA function. GABA is an inhibitory neurotransmitter.

Ethanol is absorbed into the bloodstream, mainly via the gastrointestinal tract. Effects commence within 5–10 min. The blood alcohol level peaks within 30–60 min (range 20 min to 3 hours) after last ingestion. The rate of absorption is affected by many factors, including duration of drinking, nature of drink consumed, food (and nature of the food) in the stomach, physiological factors and genetic variation. The peak ethanol concentration reached will depend on factors including gender, weight, height and rate of elimination. The rate of elimination varies within the general population from about 9 mg/100 mL blood per h to 29 mg/100 mL blood per h (median around 19 mg/100 mL per h).

DOI: 10.4324/9781003381730-11

Methanol is extremely toxic to humans, with as little as 30 mL being potentially fatal. In addition to the intoxicating effects it produces as a consequence of being a CNS depressant, similar to ethanol, methanol is metabolised to formic acid which will cause metabolic acidosis.

Medical Uses

Ethanol can be used to treat methanol poisoning.

Legal Status

The manufacture, sale and purchase of alcoholic beverages are controlled by various licensing regulations. The substance can be bought by adults aged >18 years. Offences include: being drunk in a public place; being drunk and disorderly; being drunk in charge of a child aged <7; or driving or being in charge of a vehicle, while unfit to do so through alcohol (or drugs).

Presentation and Methods of Administration

Generally it is a liquid that is taken orally. Novel, dangerous methods may sometimes be attempted, including intravenous injection and ocular absorption by, for example, pouring neat vodka into the eye with the head held back. Such practices may originate from fads on social media.

The concentration of alcohol in drink varies. Average examples are: dark spirits 40%, clear spirits 37.5%, fortified wines such as sherry 18–20%, wine 11–14%, beer 3–6%, lager 4–9%, cider 4–8%.

One unit of alcohol contains 10 mL (8 g) as pure ethanol and is approximately equivalent to half a pint of beer (alcohol by volume 3.5%), 25 mL spirits (alcohol by volume 40%) or one 100 mL glass of wine (alcohol by volume 10%).

Calculate the number of units in any drink by multiplying the total volume of a drink (in ml) by its ABV (which is measured as a percentage) and dividing the result by 1,000, e.g. 500mls of 5% lager is 2.5 units.

Guidelines set by the UK Department of Health recommend a maximum alcohol consumption of 14 units/week and that it is best spread over three days or more to minimise risks of accidents, injuries and long-term health issues. This is significantly lower than the previous recommendations.

So-called 'binge' drinking is a substantial problem, with people going out with the intention of getting very drunk. Such episodes frequently start with 'pre-loading' (sometimes known as 'prinks'), i.e. drinking cheap alcohol at home before going to pubs, clubs, or bars. This is assisted, and one might say encouraged, by the ready availability of cheap alcohol in retail outlets, particularly large supermarket stores. The consumption of numerous 'shots' of alcohol, of various types, leads to rapid alcohol absorption, which is helped by lack of food consumption, and produces a rapid rise in blood alcohol concentration. A rapid rise in blood alcohol concentration produces a greater degree of intoxication than a slower rate of increase with more noticeable intoxication even at the same blood alcohol concentration, the so-called Mellanby effect.

Alcohol is eliminated at a steady rate which is broadly equivalent to the loss of the amount of alcohol present in half a pint of average strength beer, a measure of spirits or a small glass of wine per hour.

There have been outbreaks of poisoning where home-made alcohol has been "fortified" by the addition of methanol.

Symptoms and Signs

Acute Intoxication

Physical: slurred speech, reddened conjunctivae, dilated pupils with a sluggish response to light, lateral and vertical nystagmus, loss of coordination and ataxia, rapid full-bounding pulse, increase in blood pressure and hypoglycaemia.

Psychological: stimulatory effects as a result of disinhibition of the higher brain centres, relief of tension and anxiety, relaxation and aggression may occur.

If alcohol is taken with other depressant drugs, in particular benzodiazepines, opioids or antihistamines, there is an increase in the depressant effects on the CNS with a greater risk of significant intoxication and overdose.

Methanol is poisonous and may cause blindness, coma and death. The effects may be delayed for 12–36 hours as the metabolism is slow. There may be nausea, vomiting, headache and photophobia associated with the metabolic acidosis produced via the production of formic acid.

Chronic

Signs of chronic misuse can include: a bloated, plethoric face, telangiectasia or spider naevi, reddened conjunctivae, smell of stale alcoholic liquor, acne rosacea, palmar erythema, Dupuytren's contracture, gouty tophi, obesity, gynaecomastia, striae, bruising from recurrent falls.

Many major medical complications may occur secondary to excessive alcohol over a period of years including oesophagitis, gastritis, pancreatitis, alcoholic hepatitis and cirrhosis, dementia, encephalopathy, peripheral neuropathy and myopathy, subdural haematomas, hypertension, cardiomyopathy, cardiac dysrhythmias, tuberculosis, gout, osteoporosis, and carcinoma of the oropharynx, oesophagus and liver.

Tolerance to acute intoxication develops with repeated doses and there is a strong physical dependence (see appendices for alcohol assessment questionnaires).

Withdrawal

Uncomplicated alcohol withdrawal usually occurs after 24 hours with nausea, vomiting, malaise, weakness, autonomic hyperactivity (hypertension, tachycardia, sweating, anxiety), depressed mood, irritability, transient hallucinations and illusions, headache and insomnia. See Appendix B, CIWA-Ar scale).

Delirium tremens ('DTs') starts 72–96 hours after the last alcohol ingestion with profound disorientation and confusion, with hallucinations (of any sensory modality), dilated pupils, fever, tachycardia and hypertension. There is a mortality rate of 5% and a low threshold for transfer to hospital should be observed.

Other complications include convulsions, Wernicke's encephalopathy, Korsakoff's psychosis, alcoholic hallucinosis and cardiac dysrhythmias.

Driving

The effects of alcohol on driving ability have been very well studied. The ground-breaking survey in the USA in the 1960s, the so-called 'Grand Rapids' study, demonstrated a twofold increase in the likelihood of being involved in a road traffic collision with a level of 80 mg alcohol/100 mL blood (80 mg%). The likelihood increased rapidly after this concentration and at 160 mg% the likelihood was 25-fold greater. Other studies have shown a fivefold increase in likelihood at 80 mg% and twofold at 50 mg%. Studies such as these have been used to define prescribed limits for national road traffic legislation. The UK still has a prescribed limit of 80 mg% for blood, although most other countries now have 50 mg% or 20 mg%. Some have adopted a zero tolerance approach. Full details of the UK road traffic legislation are detailed in Chapter 4.

Treatment

General: simple intoxication usually requires no treatment. Observations should be undertaken to ensure that consciousness level is not decreasing. In comatose patients general management of respiratory depression and cardiovascular collapse may be required. Treatment of hypoglycaemia may also be required.

Treatment of methanol ingestion includes the cautious administration of ethanol, treatment of acidosis and rehydration.

Withdrawal and Rehabilitation

Detoxification can be undertaken with a long-acting benzodiazepine such as chlordiazepoxide or diazepam, and there are a number of different regimens available. Detoxification should be undertaken by those with experience in the management of such patients. Disulfiram (Antabuse) is a deterrent drug, which acts by inhibiting aldehyde dehydrogenase. Unpleasant symptoms occur after a small amount of alcohol such as flushing, headache, palpitations, nausea and vomiting, and with larger doses dysrhythmias, hypertension and collapse. A card should be carried warning of the dangers of administration of alcohol because even a small amount of alcohol, such as that present in certain oral medication or mouth washes, may trigger an adverse reaction. Acamprosate calcium (Campral EC) is recommended for maintaining abstinence (the recommended treatment period is 1 year).

Other or adjunctive therapies and prevention of relapse may be assisted by counselling, intensive psychotherapy, self-help organisations (e.g. Alcoholics Anonymous) or a combination of these.

Aminoindanes, Indoles and Benzofurans

Principal Drugs and Derivatives

5, 6-Methylenedioxy-2-aminoindane, 5-methoxy-6-methyl-2-aminoindane, 2-aminoindane, 5-iodo-2-aminoindane, 5-(2-aminopropyl)-indole, 5-(2-aminopropyl)-benzofuran, 6-(2-aminopropyl)-benzofuran, MDAI gold, Pink Champagnes.

Manufacture

Illicit laboratories.

Common Street Names

MDAI, MMAI, 2-AI, 5-IAI, 5-API, 5-IT, 5-APB, 6-APB, sparkle, mindy, benzofury.

Mechanism of Action

Central nervous system stimulants although less potent than amphetamine and MDMA; may produce hallucinogenic effects. An effective dose of 5-API is 20 mg, around 150–200 mg for MDAI and 30–120 mg for 5- and 6-APB. Half-lives have not been established for humans although studies on rats suggests they are likely to be short.

Medical Uses

None, although consideration has been given to their use as an adjunct to psychotherapy.

DOI: 10.4324/9781003381730-12

Legal Status

Benzofurans are controlled by the Misuse of Drugs Act 1971 class B (from 10 June 2014).

Presentation and Methods of Administration

Powders, capsules and tablets taken orally or by snorting.

Symptoms and Signs

Acute Intoxication

Physical: dilated pupils, sweating, high blood pressure, agitation, confusion, hyperthermia.
Psychological: empathogenic effects, euphoria and intensification of sensory experiences have been reported.

Higher doses can result in irrational behaviour, confusion, fear, hallucinations, delusions, paranoia, psychosis. Deaths have been reported.

General/chronic

Unknown.

Driving

All likely to be incompatible with driving a motor vehicle but no known studies.

Treatment

Intoxication: nil – unless complications develop. Then supportive with monitoring of vital signs in hospital setting; intravenous benzodiazepines may be appropriate.

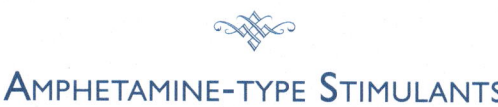

Amphetamine-type Stimulants

Principal Drugs and Derivatives

Amphetamine (Benzedrine, Adderall), dextroamphetamine (Dexedrine), fenetheylline (Captagon), lisdexamfetamine (Elvanse, Vyvanse), methamphetamine/metamphetamine/methamfetamine/metamfetamine, *p*-methoxyamphetamine (PMA), *p*-methoxymethamphetamine (PMMA), methylphenidate (Ritalin).

Manufacture

Laboratory based (legal and illegal). Methamphetamine is the most widely manufactured amphetamine-type stimulant (ATS) worldwide. There are significant public health risks from illegal production with the potential for environmental fires and accidental poisoning in clandestine laboratories. Fenetheylline is a codrug combining amphetamine with theophylline and acts as a prodrug for both components. It is produced illicitly in N. Africa and the Middle East. Lisdexamfetamine is a prodrug of d-amphetamine being combined with lysine.

Common Street Names

Amphetamine: uppers, 'A', speed, whizz, Billy whizz, wake-up, cranks, sulph, hearts, dex, dexy, dexies (Dexedrine).
Methamphetamine: crystal, ice, glass, meth.
PMA, PMMA: pink ecstasy, death, Dr Death.
Methylphenidate: diet coke, kiddie coke.

DOI: 10.4324/9781003381730-13

Mechanism of Action

Central nervous system stimulants (actions resemble those of adrenaline). When absorbed in the gastrointestinal tract they may have an effect within 20 minutes of ingestion. There is an immediate effect when injected. The effects last 4–6 h. Mostly metabolised by the liver. A substantial fraction is excreted unchanged in the urine. Half-lives lie in the range 10–30 h but may depend on urine acidity/alkalinity.

This group of drugs may be taken orally, nasally, smoked or injected intravenously (Figure 6).

Medical Uses

Amphetamine was originally used for weight reduction and as an antidepressant. It is currently used for the treatment of ADHD in children and the treatment of narcolepsy.

Lisdexamfetamine is used to treat ADHD in children but also to treat moderate to severe binge-eating disorder in adult in some countries.

Methylphenidate is used for treatment of attention deficit hyperactivity disorder (ADHD) and narcolepsy. Methamphetamine, as the l-form, is used in some formulations of 'Vicks' inhalers.

Legal Status

Amphetamine is a prescription-only medicine controlled under the Misuse of Drugs Act 1971, class B under schedule 2 (amphetamine,

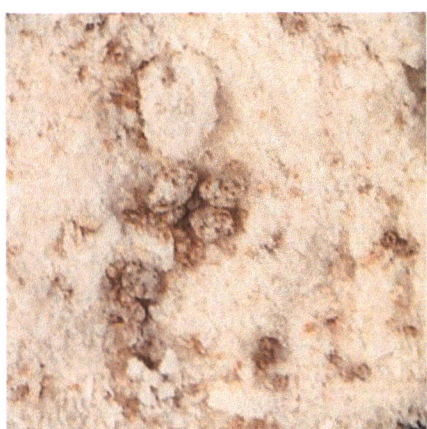

Figure 11.1 *Powder form of amphetamine.*
Source: JJ Payne-James.

dextroamphetamine, lisdexamfetamine, methylphenidate). All forms of amphetamine are class A if prepared for injection. Class A: methamphetamine, PMA, PMMA.

Presentation and Methods of Administration

Amphetamine: tablets, capsules, pale-coloured powders; base is a waxy or oily substance, sometimes with a fishy odour.
Fenetheylline: tablets.
Lisdexamfetamine: tablets.
Methamphetamine: powder or crystalline substance, also found as tablets; base is a waxy or oily substance, sometimes with a fishy odour.
Methylphenidate: tablets.
PMA, PMMA: pale-coloured powders, tablets, capsules.

Symptoms and Signs

Acute Intoxication

Physical: low-to-moderate doses (15–30 mg/24 h) result in tachypnoea, tachycardia, hypertension, loss of appetite, dilatation of pupils, brisk reflexes and fine tremor of the limbs. Higher doses will produce a dry mouth, pyrexia, sweating, blurring of vision, dizziness, bruxism, flushing or pallor, cardiac dysrhythmias and loss of coordination. These effects may last for 12 hours or more. Raised creatinine, renal failure and urinary retention have all been reported along with liver test abnormalities with a raised AST and ALT. Stereotypical behaviour – the repetition of specific acts for hours – has been reported. Pulmonary oedema and myocardial infarction have been documented. Fatalities are rarely reported but predominantly result from convulsions and intracranial haemorrhage although cardiac arrest and ventricular tachycardia, ventricular fibrillation and bradycardia have all been reported.

Methamphetamine is more prone to be injected than amphetamine, mainly due to the much higher purity sold on the street with less adulterants/bulking agents to potentially cause thrombosis.

PMA and PMMA have been reported to be particularly dangerous drugs because the stimulant effects have a slow onset of action such that the user takes more and more ('stacking') and eventually overdoses. Given the low prevalence of the drug, there is a disproportionately high incidence of death.

Psychological: euphoria, feeling of self-confidence, raised self-esteem, lowered anxiety, increased energy, greater concentration, irritability, restlessness. These perceived stimulant effects last for up to 6 hours. Higher doses can result in irrational behaviour, confusion, fear, hallucinations, delusions, paranoia and psychosis. Psychological dependence is observed although physical dependence is not generally considered to occur.

Methylphenidate is sometimes taken as a "smart pill" to enhance cognition.

When amphetamines are injected, the user additionally experiences a sensory 'rush' or 'flash', giving almost immediate sensations of enhanced energy and self-confidence and enhanced sexual enjoyment. Users rapidly develop tolerance. The 'high' reported with smoking methamphetamine is supposedly more intense than cocaine.

General/Chronic

Longer-term use requires increased dosage levels due to tolerance, with progression to intravenous use. 'Speed runs' describe the repeated use over a period of days. Several grams of amphetamines may be used daily. At the end of the 'run' the user may sleep for several days. Sometimes associated with alcohol consumption; use of cannabis or benzodiazepines may reduce anxiety caused by amphetamines. Amphetamines may be used to reduce the sedative effects of alcohol or heroin.

Physical: long-term use may additionally cause anorexia and weight loss, malnutrition, vomiting, cardiac dysrhythmias, cardiomyopathy, angina, diarrhoea, convulsions, formication, coma and death.

Psychological: in addition to the short-term effects continued amphetamine usage can cause aggression, fatigue, weakness, insomnia, anxiety, depression, suicidal ideation, and episodic, prolonged or occasionally permanent psychosis. Latent schizophrenia may be triggered by moderate use, or even by a single large dose.

Cessation/Withdrawal

Users find that cessation can cause anxiety, depression for periods of months, disturbance of sleep patterns, and irritability. Amphetamine psychosis may develop and persist for months or years after cessation.

Driving

The use of stimulant drugs can be associated with risk-taking behaviour whilst the person is experiencing the direct stimulant effects of the drug (e.g. pulling out in front of vehicles where there would normally be considered insufficient time, driving faster than normal).

Trait anger (a chronic, long-standing personality characteristic that shows up as an almost constant tendency to become angry at the slightest provocation) has been recorded as a predictor of dangerous driving behaviour amongst people who use methamphetamine.

It has been reported that acute use of amphetamine in low dosage by tired individuals can produce an improvement in attention for a short period of time, with subsequent improvement in performance of certain tasks compared with the situation in which no amphetamine has been taken. However, the effect is short-lived. Long-distance lorry drivers frequently used the drug in the 1960s and 1970s. US pilots were given low doses (5 mg) when flying long-distance missions in operations 'Desert Shield' and 'Desert Storm' in Kuwait.

It appears that amphetamine, if taken in low dosage and in the absence of other substances, may not significantly impair a person's ability to drive. In higher dosage than that associated with medical usage, the drug can impair driving ability. The after-effects of amphetamine use include poor concentration and coordination as well as drowsiness; none of these is compatible with safe driving.

Drug impairment tests are reported to perform poorly at identifying amphetamine users, with only 5% being correctly identified when low or moderate doses have been taken. Impairment is more obvious at higher doses.

Treatment

Intoxication: nil – unless complications develop. Then supportive with monitoring of vital signs in a hospital setting. Sedation and antihypertensives may be required.
General/chronic: as for intoxication.
Withdrawal: psychological support and counselling.

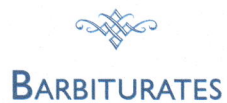

BARBITURATES

Principal Drugs

Amylobarbitone (Amytal), pentobarbital/pentobarbitone (Nembutal), quinalbarbitone (Seconal), butobarbitone (Soneryl), phenobarbital/ phenobarbitone; Tuinal contains sodium salts of amylobarbitone and quinalbarbitone.

Common Street Names

Downers, barbs, sleepers, rainbows (Tuinal), Block Busters, Christmas Trees, Goof Balls, Bluebirds, Courage pills, Downers, F-40s, Gorilla pills, Mexican yellows, Pink ladies, Reds & blues, Sleepers, Tooties, Wallbangers.

Mechanism of Action

They are sedative–hypnotic drugs that depress the central nervous system (CNS), potentiating the effects of the inhibitory neurotransmitter γ-aminobutyric acid (GABA).

Medical Uses

The intermediate-acting barbiturates should be used only for cases of severe intractable insomnia in patients already taking the drugs. Phenobarbital is used for treatment of all epileptic conditions except typical absence seizures; it is not likely to be misused. Very short-acting barbiturate drugs, such as thiopental/thiopentone, are used in anaesthesia.

DOI: 10.4324/9781003381730-14

Phenobarbital has been used in the treatment of trauma patients at high risk of alcohol withdrawal syndrome.

Legal Status

They are prescription-only medicines controlled under the Misuse of Drugs Act 1971, class B.

Presentation and Methods of Administration

Oral ingestion as tablets, capsules or elixirs; can be injected as a liquid preparation from an injection vial. Most barbiturates are very rarely encountered since the introduction of benzodiazepines (fewer than 10,000 prescriptions for barbiturates other than phenobarbital in England in 2012). Phenobarbital is still regularly prescribed.

Symptoms and Signs

Acute Intoxication

Physical: Clinical effects are predominantly central nervous signs and symptoms including confusion, slurred speech, ataxia, diplopia, horizontal nystagmus, somnolence and coma. Can cause cardiovascular depression and vasodilation, leading to hypotension, cardiovascular collapse, hypothermia, and multisystem organ failure. Ileus may occur due to gastrointestinal depression. Nausea and vomiting are also commonly seen in barbiturate intoxication. For most of the more powerful barbiturates there is a narrow margin between therapeutic and lethal doses. The risks of complications from injection are increased because they are poorly water soluble.

Psychological: anxiolytic, impairment of memory and cognition.

Chronic

Sedative–hypnotic drugs cause physical and psychological dependence and an abstinence syndrome. Chronic intoxication occurs because there is an upper limit to tolerance with sedative–hypnotic drugs and individuals often increase their regular consumption above this point.

There may be nystagmus, difficulty with accommodation and ataxia, and with higher doses drowsiness, coma and death.

Withdrawal starts within 24 hours with anxiety, tremor, insomnia, restlessness and tachycardia; blood pressure, respiration rate and temperature may be slightly raised. Fits may occur, especially with persistent tachycardia (>100 beats/min).

Driving

As most barbiturates produce profound CNS depression, driving while taking the drugs is not recommended. Phenobarbital is unlikely to produce significant adverse effects although normal guidelines relating to epilepsy and driving apply.

Treatment

There is cross-tolerance between the different barbiturates, and therefore any barbiturate can be used to treat the withdrawal syndrome of another. Benzodiazepines may also be used.

If dependent on prescribed drugs, gradual reduction over several weeks or months may be possible. If large doses are used it may be more appropriate that detoxification should be carried out in hospital.

Treatment should be aimed at preventing the medical complications of fits and psychosis with a long-acting benzodiazepine such as diazepam.

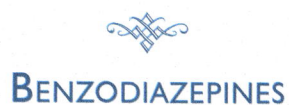

Benzodiazepines

Principal Drugs

Diazepam (Valium), temazepam (Normison), lorazepam (Ativan), oxazepam (Serenid), nitrazepam (Mogadon), chlordiazepoxide (Librium), clonazepam (Rivotril), flunitrazepam (Rohypnol), midazolam (Hypnovel), alprazolam (Xanax), triazolam (Halcion), etizolam (Etilaam, Sedekopan). Numerous new 'designer' benzodiazepines including phenazepam, flualprazolam, flubromazolam, flubromazepam.

Common Street Names

All: benzos, nerve pills.
Diazepam: (Figure 7) vallies, blues, yellows.
Temazepam: jellies, eggs, temazzies.
Nitrazepam: moggies.
Chlordiazepoxide: tranxies.
Flunitrazepam: roofies.
Alprazolam: Upjohns.
Phenazepam: Russian Valium.

Mechanism of Action

These sedative–hypnotic drugs depress the central nervous system (CNS). The benzodiazepine group of drugs produces their pharmacological effects by enhancing λ-aminobutyric acid (GABA) transmission; consequently abrupt cessation of the drugs will result in a reduction in GABA function. GABA is an inhibitory neurotransmitter.

DOI: 10.4324/9781003381730-15

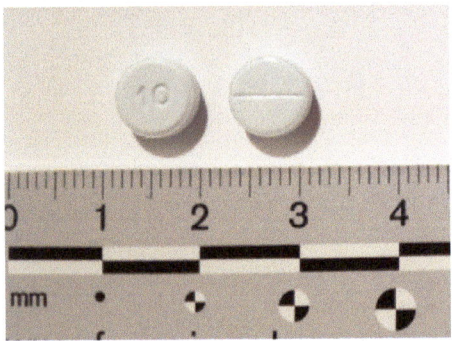

Figure 13.1 *Two 10 mg tablets of diazepam.*
Source: JJ Payne-James.

Benzodiazepines (BZs) are classified as very short acting (e.g. midazolam half-life of 2.5 h), short acting (e.g. temazepam half-life 10–17 h), intermediate acting (e.g. diazepam half-life 30–60 h) and long acting (e.g. flurazepam half-life 50–100 h). Hypnotic benzodiazepines would normally be taken at night before retiring to bed. Others are prescribed according to the condition being treated and may be taken several times a day in divided doses.

Most benzodiazepines are extensively metabolised and some metabolites are themselves pharmacologically active also.

Medical Uses

Benzodiazepines are used as anxiolytic and sedative drugs. They are also useful for the treatment of muscle spasm (e.g. as adjuncts to analgesia in acute back pain). Some benzodiazepines such as clonazepam may be used in the treatment of epilepsy.

Diazepam and others may be used as a premedication before surgery or other diagnostic procedures.

Many of the benzodiazepines are subject to non-prescription use (abuse), often in higher than recommended dosages.

Legal Status

Many BZs are prescription-only medicines controlled under the Misuse of Drugs Act, class C and under the Misuse of Drugs Regulations 1985, schedule 4 (except temazepam and flunitrazepam, which are in schedule 3, making it an offence to possess the drug without a prescription). New BZs fall within the new Psychoactive Substances Act 2016.

The product licence for triazolam was suspended in the UK in 1991 because of adverse side effects, including a higher incidence of psychiatric disturbances.

Presentation and Methods of Administration

Tablets, oral and injection solutions; suppositories. Normally taken orally or injected.

Benzodiazepines are increasingly encountered in combination with opioids such as heroin, fentanyl and occasionally nitazenes, particularly in N. America (benzo dope).

Symptoms and Signs

Acute Intoxication

Physical: dizziness, sedation, loss of coordination, weight gain and sexual dysfunction. High doses (overdose) may result in low blood pressure and coma. Death is unusual with benzodiazepines.

Psychological: relief of anxiety, promotion of relaxation, memory impairment. There may be a 'paradoxical' behavioural response with increased aggression and hostility.

Uncharacteristic events may occur: shoplifting, self-exposure, or uncontrollable emotional responses such as giggling or weeping.

There is a 'hangover' effect even in low dosage. The following day there may be drowsiness, inability to concentrate and impairment of tasks such as driving or operating machinery. Phenazepam may cause extreme sedation for 2–3 days.

Alcohol and benzodiazepines increase each other's actions and marked impairment can occur. The CNS depressant effects of other drugs, including analgesics, antidepressants and antihistamines, may be enhanced. The MHRA/CHM provide advice regarding the use of benzodiazepines and opioids, for example (March 2020 https://bnf.nice. org.uk/drugs/diazepam/#indications-and-dose).

Chronic

Tolerance develops rapidly to both the sedative and the anxiolytic effects. There is cross-tolerance for the BZs, alcohol and other non-barbiturate hypnotics, including chlormethiazole.

Physical and psychological dependence occurs with chronic intoxication in those who regularly take large doses.

Chronic intoxication occurs because there is an upper limit to tolerance to sedative–hypnotic drugs and dependent individuals increase their daily consumption beyond this. The clinical manifestations are not unlike alcohol intoxication, with slurred speech, difficulty in concentration, poor comprehension, memory impairment, emotional liability with irritability and depressed mood.

Withdrawal symptoms occur in 20–40% of long-term users who have received therapeutic doses for 4–6 months. Symptoms may occur within 2–3 days of stopping the short-acting drugs and within 7–10 days of stopping the longer-acting drugs.

The withdrawal syndrome results in: anxiety, sweating, insomnia, headache, tremor, nausea; disordered perceptions including feelings of unreality, abnormal bodily sensations, hypersensitivity to stimuli; psychosis and convulsions.

Driving

Many studies have been undertaken investigating the effects of benzodiazepines on driving. Generally, it has been found that, when first taken, or if taken in inappropriate dosage, the effects of benzodiazepine drugs on driving ability can be significant. Reaction times are slowed, visual perception may be impaired and time to process information can be increased, all leading to poor driving. There is a significant increase in road traffic collisions. Lack of coordination and slurred speech may be apparent. Tolerance may develop if the drugs are taken daily and thereafter the effects on driving ability may be small.

Treatment

Intoxication: mainly supportive because BZs have a high toxic–therapeutic ratio. Flumazenil is a specific benzodiazepine antagonist that produces rapid reversal of sedation; however, it should not be used in the pre-hospital care environment because of the risk of mixed overdoses with complications such as seizures and dysrhythmias.

Withdrawal: change to a long-acting benzodiazepine such as diazepam and reduce dose over a period of time. High-dose dependency may require in-patient detoxification. The risk of seizures is greater with high-dose dependency.

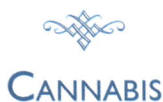

CANNABIS

Principal Drugs

Cannabis is the common name for the plant *Cannabis sativa* (Figures 8a, 8b), which contains a large number of active compounds known collectively as cannabinoids, the most important, and active, of which is known as delta-9-tetrahydrocannabinol (Δ^9-THC). Another important cannabinoid is cannabidiol (CBD). Cannabis is a mild sedative, which is used for its euphoric and relaxing properties. It is the most widely misused controlled drug in the UK.

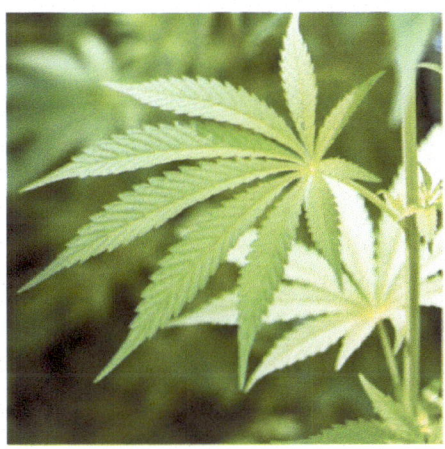

Figure 14.1 *(a) Cannabis leaf*
Source: Shutterstock.

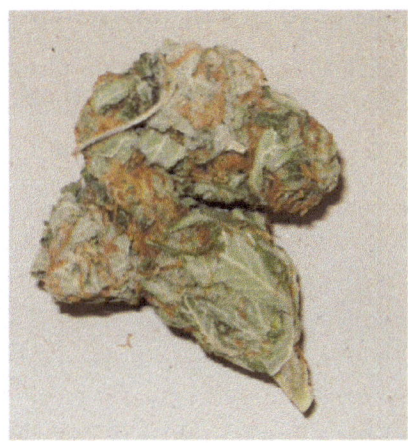

Figure 14.1 *(b) dried cannabis fruiting material ('bud')*
Source: JJ Payne-James.

DOI: 10.4324/9781003381730-16

Manufacture

Most cannabis used currently is in the form of the herbal material, rather than the previously widely used cannabis resin. Most herbal cannabis is now grown within the UK, often in large quantities amounting to commercial production. Such production may use sophisticated growing conditions, which can be on an industrial scale in warehouses, although in recent years converted lofts, garages or other rooms are more frequently encountered. Such outfits will normally use a means of bypassing the electricity meter because they use large amounts of energy. Extraction filters are also often used to remove the characteristic odour. The plants are normally cuttings taken from a mother plant and are therefore genetically identical and often grown in a fibrous medium without soil (hydroponics).

Common Street Names

Pot, dope, blow, grass, marijuana, ganja, nabis, weed, hash, hashish, draw, puff, skunk, sinsemilla, green, hemp.

Mechanism of Action

THC is absorbed rapidly in the lungs and the plasma concentration peaks quickly, within a few minutes, although peak effects occur later at about 15–30 mins and last for 2–4 h. If ingested orally the onset of action is slower, although the effects last longer, perhaps up to 8 h. THC is very fat soluble and rapidly deposited in fatty tissue around the body. Consequently, THC may leak out of fat into the bloodstream over a long period of time after the last use. If a regular, heavy user of the drug abstains for a period, cannabis use may still be detectable in the blood for many days and in urine for weeks afterwards.

THC breaks down in the body to THC-COOH (carboxy-THC), which is inactive, via 11-OH-THC (hydroxy-THC), which is pharmacologically active. There are hundreds of other cannabinoids present within the material, including cannabidiol (CBD) and cannabinol (CBN). Home-grown strains of cannabis may contain THC at a concentration in excess of 30% when harvested, although the normal value may be closer to around 10–15% THC; however, this is still much stronger than foreign imported cannabis which is normally of THC strength 3–4%.

There is increasing evidence that another cannabinoid, CBD, may moderate some of the less pleasant effects of THC. Typical herbal cannabis contains THC and CBD, whereas some of the specially bred varieties, often referred to as 'skunk' on account of the potent odour, may contain THC with only minimal or no CBD. This may account for the increasingly reported adverse effects after heavy cannabis ('skunk') use.

Since around 2020 other isomers of Δ^9-THC have been encountered, the main one of which is Δ^8-THC. This compound has similar, but less pronounced effects, than Δ^9-THC.

The ninth report of the UK House of Lords Science and Technology Committee (1998) defined categories of cannabis users:

- A *casual user* may be defined as someone who is an irregular cannabis user, smoking amounts of up to 1 g at a time but not more than 28 g/year.
- A *regular user* can be defined as smoking 0.5 g/day in three to four joints (i.e. about 150 mg cannabis per cigarette), adding up to about 3.5 g/week.
- A *heavy user* can be defined as smoking more than 3.5 g/day and ≥28 g/week. This group Heavy and regular users are sometimes referred to as 'stoners' is likely to be more or less permanently intoxicated – 'stoned'.

Medical Uses

Cannabis products may help symptoms such as muscle spasm in patients with multiple sclerosis and the nausea and vomiting induced by chemotherapy. Many users claim that it has analgesic properties. Some medicinal preparations have been licensed for restricted use in many countries including, for example, the UK and the USA for treating conditions such as mentioned above (THC) but also for severe forms of epilepsy (CBD). Research is on-going into many other possible uses of THC, CBD and other cannabinoids.

Legal Status

Cannabis is a controlled drug under the Misuse of Drugs Act 1971. It is illegal to grow, possess or supply the drug. The Home Office can grant a licence for special purposes such as research. Herbal cannabis (except seeds and stalks), cannabis resin and cannabis oil are classified as class B drugs.

'Cannabis-based products for medicinal use in humans' ('CBPM') is a defined category of cannabis, cannabis resin, cannabinol and cannabinol derivatives – listed in schedule 2 to the MDR 2001 and removed from designation under the 2015 Order.

Presentation and Methods of Administration

Forms of cannabis include herbal material, resin and honey-oil. Cannabis resin is a concentrated form of the herbal material, made with those parts of the plant that contain the greatest concentration of the active component; this is preferentially removed and formed into hard blocks. The THC component of cannabis may also be concentrated by extraction into so-called 'honey-oil'. This particular practice has caused many injuries and even fatalities.

The drug is normally used by smoking in the form of a cigarette, commonly referred to as a 'reefer', 'joint', 'spliff' or 'blunt'; vaping is also popular. The drug can also be smoked via a pipe, sometimes an elaborate construction referred to as a 'bong', and is occasionally taken orally in the form of cakes or other fat-containing food, which allows the THC to be extracted from the cannabis (e.g. chocolate, cookies).

Symptoms and Signs

The exact effects of cannabis are reported to depend on the amount used, the social setting, and the user's expectations and previous experience with the drug. Cannabis is usually smoked with effects starting within seconds, peaking between 15 and 30 min, and lasting for 2 h or so. Occasionally effects may last up to 4 h. However, this will also depend on factors such as the number and depth of inhalations from each 'joint' smoked.

Acute Intoxication

Physical: dryness of the mouth, hunger ('munchies'), reddened conjunctivae, increased blood pressure associated with postural hypotension and tachycardia, with slight impairment of psychomotor and cognitive function.

Psychological: a feeling of wellbeing, euphoria, and increased self-confidence, relaxation; perceptions, e.g. smell, taste and hearing may be enhanced. There may be poor concentration, memory impairment, suggestibility and difficulty with tasks requiring manual dexterity. Occasionally anxiety, agitation and paranoia or a toxic psychosis may occur. Flashbacks may occur after the effects of the drugs wear off, more commonly when other drugs such as LSD have been used as well. The effects from the more potent home-grown varieties are likely to be more intense and may last for longer than non-'skunk' varieties.

Chronic

Before the appearance of 'skunk' cannabis there was little clear evidence that cannabis use caused physical or mental-health problems in the long term. More recently there have been increasing numbers of mental-health problems identified.

Cannabis psychosis may occur after consumption of a large quantity of cannabis or following frequent consumption of high-potency forms of the drug. Confusion occurs suddenly, and is associated with delusions, hallucinations and emotional lability.

There may be temporary amnesia with disorientation, depersonalisation and paranoia. There may also be a cannabis-induced functional psychosis, which responds swiftly to antipsychotic medication, but tends to relapse with resumption of cannabis usage.

High-dose chronic use may result in reduced testosterone and sperm count, reduced fertility in women and premature birth, with a corresponding reduction in fetal birthweight.

There may be an effect on the immune system, making users more susceptible to bacterial infections. There have been suggestions that prolonged use of cannabis may lead to brain damage but there is no conclusive evidence for this. Frequent inhalation of cannabis smoke over a long period may result in respiratory problems such as bronchitis and perhaps lung cancer (although this may relate in part to concurrent tobacco usage).

Tolerance develops rapidly within a few days of regular drug use and decays rapidly when drug use ceases. With very heavy use physical dependence may occur, with a mild abstinence syndrome starting a few hours after stopping the drug and lasting for 4–5 days.

Withdrawal can result in irritability, restlessness, decreased appetite and weight loss.

Driving

Studies have shown that THC impairs driving in a dose-related manner. Maximum impairment after cannabis use is seen around 30–45 min after smoking, with the effects dissipating over the next 2–3 h.

Effects produced by cannabis relevant to driving can include a slowing of decision-making and reaction time, impairment of ability to maintain road positioning, impairment of ability to perform tasks requiring divided attention, impaired peripheral vision, lack of concentration and fatigue. Some drivers may compensate for this by driving more slowly and a not infrequent scenario is for a driver to be brought to the attention of the police by driving very slowly.

Significant impairment of driving performance would not normally be expected to be observed for more than 1–2 h after use. Cannabis use would not normally be expected to be associated with risk-taking activities.

The prevalence of the involvement of cannabis in road traffic collisions and fatalities is unclear, due to the rapid breakdown of THC in the body and its instability in vitro once a blood sample has been taken.

Treatment

There is no specific treatment.

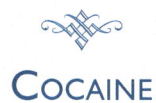

COCAINE

This is an alkaloid derived from the leaves of the coca bush (*Erythroxylon coca*) which grows predominantly in South America but to a lesser extent in Africa, the Far East and India.

Principal Drugs and Derivatives

Cocaine hydrochloride, cocaine base, crack. A number of synthetic 'caines' appeared for sale via the internet in the early 2010s, including dimethocaine and 4-fluorotropacocaine, but appear to have fallen out of favour.

Manufacture

It is refined through a number of purification stages in illegal factories from leaves to paste to cocaine hydrochloride.

Common Street Names

Coke, 'C', charlie, wash, nose-candy, crack, rock, snow, stone, oxi, oxi-dado. Synthetic 'caines' have been referred to by the street names mind melt, amplify, mania and stardust.

Mechanism of Action

As a central nervous system (CNS) stimulant cocaine blocks reuptake of dopamine and, to a lesser extent, noradrenaline and serotonin. It is metabolised primarily to benzoylecgonine and ecgonine methyl ester in

DOI: 10.4324/9781003381730-17

the liver. Some cocaine (20%) is excreted unchanged in the urine. The half-life of cocaine is 0.7–1.5 h, that of benzoylecgonine 5–8 h. Benzoylecgonine may be detected for several days after last use. The onset of action, half-life and duration of effects depend on the route of administration. When sniffed/snorted, the effects are felt within a few minutes and last up to a maximum of an hour; doses may have to be repeated every 20 min. If smoked or injected the effects are immediate and last 15–30 min. A typical abuse dose is around 100–200mg.

Cocaine may be subject to repeated use (bingeing) which can last many hours or even a day or two during which much larger amounts of cocaine are used.

The stimulant effects last longer, but are less intense, and the comedown is somewhat moderated if used together with alcohol. Rebound sedation (a 'crash') may be noted due to neurotransmitter depletion.

Medical Uses

Cocaine was used as a surface anaesthetic (e.g. in ear/nose/throat surgery) but this is now rare.

Legal Status

Cocaine is a prescription-only medicine, class A under schedule 2 of the Misuse of Drugs Act 1971. The synthetic 'caines' fall within the Psychoactive Substances Act 2016.

Presentation and Methods of Administration

Ear, nose and throat surgery as an oromucosal solution (10%) or nasal spray.
Illicit cocaine can be encountered in various forms including:
Coca leaf: normally chewed or made into an infusion ('coca tea') although such use is uncommon outside the countries of origin.
White crystals/powder (cocaine hydrochloride): may be snorted through a straw or rolled-up paper, e.g. bank note in 'lines', or from a small 'coke spoon', or may be injected into veins or applied to mucous membranes (e.g. mouth/rectum/vagina). Cocaine hydrochloride purity can vary widely but is often in the range 50–80%. Concurrent use with alcohol is widespread.

'Crack', base, paste: cocaine hydrochloride powder may be basified to produce 'crack' (Figure 9), which can be a potent form of cocaine, by mixing it with baking soda and heating. The product is variable in appearance – as white or yellow, small, waxy-looking lumps that may be smoked in cigarettes or pipe; it may also be mixed with heroin and injected ('snowballing' or 'speedballing'). Special water pipes are used by some to prevent destruction of the smoked drug by high temperatures. Homemade pipes can be made from a variety of readily available items such as glass or plastic bottles and silver foil.

Synthetic 'caines': normally encountered as white powders and are taken via snorting.

Symptoms and Signs

Acute Intoxication

Physical: the effects are short acting, but dose dependent. The user may experience tachycardia, sweating, significant pupillary dilatation, hyper-pyrexia, reduced appetite, reduced need for sleep or formication. It can present as acute behavioural disturbance (ABD) (see Chapter 5). Death

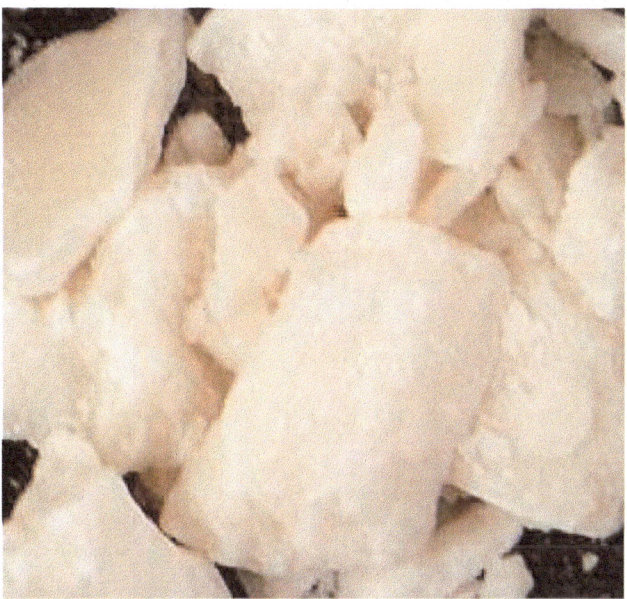

Figure 15.1 *Crack cocaine.*
Source: JJ Payne-James.

may occur rapidly secondary to convulsion, intracranial haemorrhage, respiratory arrest or cardiac arrhythmias. The risk of an adverse event is increased if used together with alcohol, resulting in the formation of cocaethylene which has greater cardiotoxicity.

Psychological: euphoria, sensation of increased physical and mental well-being; these may be followed by irritability, depression and insomnia; paranoia may develop. A greater propensity towards violence has been reported for the combination of crack cocaine with alcohol.

General/chronic

Physical: in addition to the above effects, chest pains and muscle spasms may occur. Impotence and failure of ejaculation have been reported in men, and difficulty in achieving orgasm in women. Rhinorrhoea (runny nose), eczema localised around the nose and nasal septum damage (erosions, necrosis, perforations) with anosmia can develop. Weight loss and malnutrition are common.

Psychological: as for acute intoxication. Tolerance develops. A heavy cocaine user may ingest up to several grams daily. Disturbance of eating and sleeping patterns may occur.

Cessation/Withdrawal

It is now generally accepted that physical and marked psychological dependence occurs. This is manifest with muscle pains and tremor, hunger, irritability, depression, fatigue and prolonged sleep episodes, which can last for 24 hours or more. Psychological dependence with craving and intense drug-seeking behaviour occurs. A severe withdrawal syndrome known as 'the crash' occurs.

Driving

The use of stimulant drugs can be associated with risk-taking while the person is experiencing the direct stimulant effects of the drug (e.g. pulling out in front of vehicles when normally there would be insufficient time, driving faster than normal). However, with cocaine these stimulant effects last for only a short period of time, after which the after-effects start. It has been reported that acute (i.e. one-off) use of cocaine by tired individuals can produce an improvement in attention for a short period of time, with subsequent improvement in performance of simple tasks. As the tasks become more complex, however, this improvement may not occur.

The after-effects of cocaine use include poor concentration and coordination as well as drowsiness, all of which are not compatible with safe driving. Lapses of attention and ignoring stimuli such as changing traffic lights have been reported by all users in one study.

Some cocaine users report disturbances in their peripheral vision ('snow lights'), which distract attention; visual impairment, primarily caused by an increased sensitivity to light, has been reported by many users, presumably due to the pupillary dilatation produced by cocaine.

The studies performed investigating the effects of cocaine on driving have been limited by the dosages permitted because only low-dose studies have been authorised, given the dangers associated with cocaine use.

A study of cocaine-dependent individuals showed a slower reaction time than in non-dependent individuals, which was still evident 3 months after drug cessation.

Drug impairment tests are reported to perform poorly in identifying cocaine users, with almost half of such users performing 'normally' on such tests when prior cocaine use had been established via laboratory testing of urine specimens.

Treatment

Intoxication

Nil unless complications develop. Then treatment is supportive with monitoring of vital signs in a hospital setting, using fluids, cooling and sedation as required, together with treatment of complications such as seizures, coronary syndromes and arrhythmias as they occur.

General/Chronic

As for intoxication.

Withdrawal

This needs psychological support and counselling, including treatment of depression and sleep disturbance.

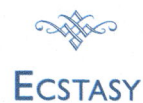

ECSTASY

Principal Drugs

3,4-Methylenedioxymethamphetamine (MDMA), 3,4-methylenedioxy-ethamphetamine(MDEA), 3,4-methylenedioxyamphetamine (MDA). Some other similar compounds may also be referred to as 'ecstasy' including PMA and PMMA for which see 'Amphetamine-type Stimulants'.

These drugs (Figure 10) are used recreationally, typically in club and dance culture, for their central stimulant and psychedelic properties resulting in euphoria, and dissociative and empathogenic effects.

Manufacture

Laboratory/factory production.

Common Street Names

Ecstasy, E, XTC, doves, Dennis, Adam (MDMA), Eve (MDEA) Molly, E-bomb, hug drug, Scooby snacks, Smarties.

Mechanism of Action

These drugs are powerful central nervous system (CNS) stimulants with mild hallucinogenic properties. MDMA acts predominantly on presynaptic 5-hydroxytryptamine 2 ($5HT_2$) receptors and increases the activity of serotonin, dopamine, and noradrenaline. Compared with the very potent stimulant methamphetamine, MDMA causes greater serotonin release and somewhat lesser dopamine release. Serotonin is a

DOI: 10.4324/9781003381730-18

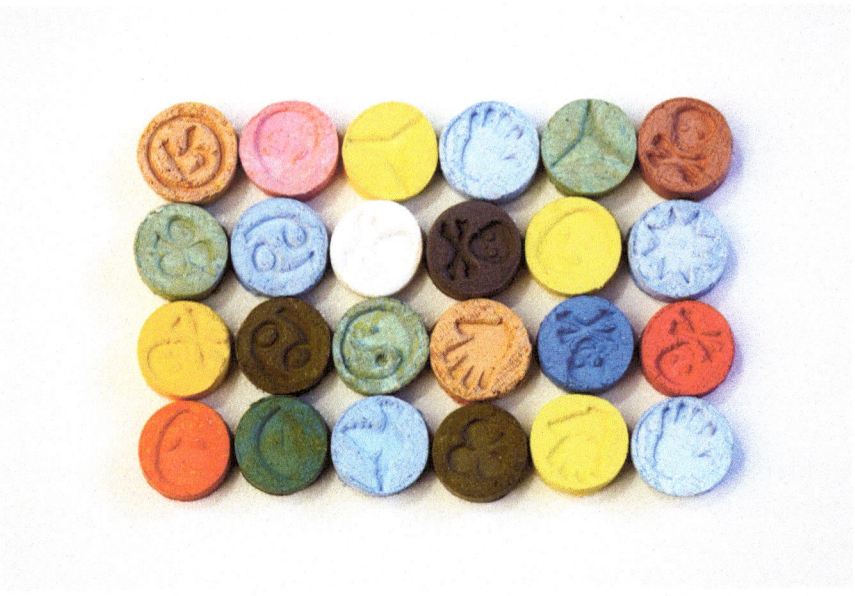

Figure 16.1 *Examples of MDMA.*
Source: Shutterstock

neurotransmitter that plays an important role in the regulation of mood, sleep, pain, emotion, appetite and other behaviours. The excess release of serotonin by MDMA is most probably responsible for the elevation of mood. However, by releasing large amounts of serotonin, MDMA causes the brain to become significantly depleted of this important neurotransmitter, contributing to the negative behavioural after-effects that users often experience for several days after taking MDMA.

Medical Uses

Nil. MDMA was previously used in psychotherapeutic settings.

Legal Status

Class A under schedule 2 of the Misuse of Drugs Act 1971 (1977 Modification Order).

Presentation and Methods of Administration

Tablets, which are of variable colours, frequently with a logo (e.g. dove, Mitsubishi, smiley face, star), capsules and crystalline powders; the latter are often of high purity. Dosages are difficult to quantify owing to the large range of synthetic byproducts and additives often used in preparation (e.g. caffeine, amphetamine analogues, ketamine). Powders in particular are prone to produce overdosage due to their frequent high purity. Some tablets have been found to contain large, excessive amounts of MDMA. Occasionally tablets sold as containing MDMA do not contain any of the drug at all. MDEA is currently rarely encountered. Generally, ecstasy is taken by mouth, and only very rarely injected, snorted or smoked. Co-ingestion with alcohol is now frequent.

Symptoms and Signs

Acute Intoxication

Physical: effects take up to 1 hour to appear after ingestion and may last for several hours. These are dose dependent – a moderate dose being between 75 and 100 mg; symptoms include tachycardia, dry mouth and throat, jaw clenching and grinding, sweating, pyrexia, nausea and vomiting, transient anorexia, loss of coordination, headache, fatigue, trismus, nystagmus, blurring of vision, ataxia, muscle cramps, urinary urgency, brisk reflexes and paraesthesia.

In overdose or in susceptible individuals, convulsions, hyper- or hypotension, severe hyperthermia, cardiac dysrhythmias, disseminated intravascular coagulation, rhabdomyolysis and renal failure have been reported. These symptoms are caused by excessive amounts of serotonin (serotonin syndrome). Deaths have been reported in association with the use of single tablets (not caused by contaminants, as has been suggested). Some deaths have been related to cerebral oedema (secondary to excess water ingestion) since the drug has an antidiuretic effect on the kidney. The effects may be exacerbated or precipitated by associated physical activity, e.g. dancing in a hot environment within a club. The toxic effects of MDMA may be enhanced with alcohol.

Psychological: a mild, euphoric 'rush', feelings of energy and vitality, increased self-esteem, increased self-confidence, feeling of empathy with others, visual and auditory hallucinations (rarely unpleasant); flashbacks may occur, and anxiety attacks, aggression, insomnia or psychosis.

General/chronic

Physical: as for acute intoxication. Physical dependence is not generally considered to occur, although tolerance does occur. Liver abnormalities have been reported. Impairment of cognitive ability has been reported. *Psychological:* as for acute intoxication. Flashbacks may be increasingly experienced. Psychological dependence is not believed to occur. Recreational use of ecstasy is associated with significant deficits in neurocognitive function (particularly immediate and delayed verbal memory) and increased psychopathological symptoms.

Cessation/Withdrawal

After the acute effects of the drug have worn off, the user may experience several days of anxiety, depression and fatigue, variously described as a 'weekend high followed by a midweek low'. Rebound effects include exhaustion, apathy, depression, irritability and insomnia.

Driving

The initial stimulant effects typically last up to 4 h with residual after-effects lasting up to 12 h or more, or often until the person has slept. The stimulant effects, which are very similar to those produced by amphetamine, include increased wakefulness, increased self-confidence and a feeling of physical wellbeing. The reported side or adverse effects include thirst and dilated pupils of the eyes.

The after-effects of the drug are reported to include physical exhaustion, drowsiness, anxiety, agitation and disorientation, which may last for 48 h or more after ingestion of the drug.

The use of stimulant drugs can be associated with risk-taking while the person is experiencing the direct stimulant effects of the drug, e.g. pulling out in front of vehicles where there would normally be insufficient time to do so or driving faster than normal. It has, however, been reported that acute use of stimulant drugs in low dosage by tired individuals can produce an improvement in attention for a short period of time, with subsequent improvement in performance of certain tasks compared with the situation where no drug has been taken. However, the effect is short-lived.

It is reported that basic vehicle control is only moderately affected. There are, however, indications that under the influence of MDMA individuals accept higher levels of risk. Others have concluded that MDMA use should be considered inconsistent with safe driving immediately following ingestion and for up to a day or longer following use.

Treatment

Intoxication: close observation of pulse rate, blood pressure, temperature, and mental state. If any of these are abnormal, observation should be within a hospital setting where facilities for supportive treatment (e.g. ventilation, intracranial pressure monitoring) are readily available. Serotonin syndrome is a possibility, especially if another drug producing serotonin, or preventing reuptake, is ingested. Treatment with benzodiazepines and i/v fluids may be appropriate.

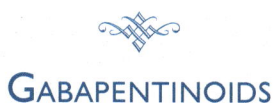

GABAPENTINOIDS

Principal Drugs

Gabapentin (Neurontin), pregabalin (Lyrica).

Common Street Names

Gabapentin: gabbies, johnnies.
Pregabalin: Budweisers, buds.

Mechanism of Action

Gabapentin and pregabalin are sedative–hypnotic drugs which have depressant effects on the central nervous system (CNS). Both are analogs of gamma-aminobutyric acid (GABA) but are not thought to act on GABA receptors, instead acting selectively via the α-2-δ subunit of the N-type calcium channel. Ultimately this results in a decrease in the release of glutamate and noradrenaline.

The half-lives for both are relatively short (5–9 h gabapentin, 5–6.5 h pregabalin). Neither drug undergoes significant metabolism with the parent drug being by far the most abundant compound excreted in urine (80–90%).

Medical Uses

Gabapentinoids are used to treat epilepsy, generalized anxiety disorder (pregabalin), as an adjunct for partial seizures and for neuropathic pain, postherpetic neuralgia, diabetic peripheral neuropathy and fibromyalgia.

DOI: 10.4324/9781003381730-19

Gabapentinoids are also subject to abuse, often in higher than recommended dosages and particularly by the opiate-using population and can produce relaxation and limited euphoria and risks of fatality. Dissociative and entactogenic effects have also been reported. Pregabalin is thought to be more liable to abuse than gabapentin due to possessing greater potency, a faster onset of action (1 h vs 3–4 h) and a higher bioavailability.

Legal Status

Gabapentin and pregabalin are prescription-only medicines controlled under the Misuse of Drugs Act, class C and under the Misuse of Drugs Regulations 1985, schedule 3.

Presentation and Methods of Administration

Tablets. Normally taken orally or injected. Occasional snorting when abused.

Symptoms and Signs

Acute intoxication

Physical: dizziness, sedation, loss of coordination, loss of consciousness (rare).
Psychological: anxiety, depression, suicidal ideation, difficulty sleeping.

Chronic

Physical and psychological dependence occurs with chronic intoxication in those who regularly take large (excessive) doses.

Although the bioavailability of gabapentin falls from 60% to 33% with an increase in dosage from 900mg/day to 3,600mg/day, that for pregabalin stays high (>90%) and is independent of dosage. Tolerance develops rapidly to both the sedative and the anxiolytic effects.

Symptoms may occur within 12 h to 7 days of ceasing medication. For those taking the drugs for seizure disorders there is a significant risk of seizures returning.

Withdrawal symptoms include: anxiety, insomnia, headache, nausea, dizziness, aches/pain, irritability, restlessness.

Driving

If taken according to prescription gabapentinoids would not be expected to produce adverse effects on driving ability. If taken to excess, or in combination with other psychoactive drugs as is a frequent occurrence, both could contribute to production of impairing effects.

Treatment

Intoxication: little required due to high toxic–therapeutic ratio when taken alone and the main effect being only mild sedation. Treatment should be focused on any co-ingested compounds, if required.

Withdrawal: reduce dose over a period of time. High-dose dependency may require in-patient detoxification. The risk of seizures is greater with high-dose dependency.

γ-Hydroxybutyrate and Related Compounds

Principal Drugs

γ-Hydroxybutyrate (GHB); γ-butyrolactone (GBL); 1,4-butanediol (BD).

Common Street Names

GHB: liquid E, liquid X, liquid ecstasy, easylay, GBH, grievous bodily harm, Georgia home boy, salt water, circles, date rape drug, forget pill, forget-me pill, La Rocha

GBL: blue nitro, gamma BL, miracle clean, midnight blue, paint stripper, wax stripper, video cleaner.

BD: Pine needle oil/extract, miracle cleaning products, herbal GHB.

All three drugs are chemically closely related. GHB and GBL can be interconverted by simply changing the acidity or alkalinity of the solution.

The observed effects of all three substances are indistinguishable.

Mechanism of Action

They are anaesthetic with a sedative rather than an analgesic effect. GHB is a naturally occurring substance related structurally to GABA (γ-aminobutryic acid) and may be an inhibitory neurotransmitter.

Effects commence between 10 min and an hour after ingestion; if taken in high dosage the effects may last for several hours. Peak plasma levels are achieved within an hour; the drugs have a very short half-life of only 20–60 min or so and, due to their chemical structures, are rarely part of routine drug-testing or drug screening procedures. Specific

DOI: 10.4324/9781003381730-20

procedures will be able to detect the drugs only up to a few hours in blood and perhaps up to 8–12 h in urine.

Medical Uses

GHB has been used as a premedicant and, in the UK as the sodium salt, sodium oxybate (Xyrem), to treat narcolepsy with associated cataplexy. GBL and BD have no medical uses.

Legal Status

In 2021 GHB, GBL and BD were moved from class C to class B under the Misuse of Drugs Act 1971 following a number of high-profile cases.

Presentation and Methods of Administration

Sodium oxybate: oral solution 500 mg/mL.
Illicit: colourless liquids often sold in small bottles. GBL has a chemical/solvent odour. GHB may also be available as powder or in capsules, however it rapidly absorbs water to become damp and sticky. The strength of liquids can vary greatly from virtually pure to much less so. GHB is often sold in a clear liquid at around 20% purity. It is taken orally, often as spoon- or capfuls, rarely injected; the drug may sometimes be inserted into the anus. Although implicated in drug-facilitated sexual assaults the drug has rarely been detected in such cases. The drugs are used widely within the club and dance scene and by body builders as GHB is reported to influence growth hormone levels.

Symptoms and Signs

Acute Intoxication

Physical effects depend on the dose taken. At low-to-moderate dosage (1–2 g) there is euphoria initially, then sedation, nausea and vomiting, profuse sweating, stiffening of muscles and disorientation; at higher doses (upwards of 2 g) there is ataxia, convulsions, delirium, visual disturbances, coma, bradycardia, hypotension, Cheyne–Stokes respiration and respiratory collapse. The effects can wear off very quickly, although 'hangover' effects may persist for longer. There is a narrow margin between euphoric intoxication and coma, and the effects are worse when mixed with other central nervous system depressants, especially alcohol.

Long-term Effects

Unknown, but physical and psychological dependence may occur. Withdrawal effects include anxiety, delirium, confusion, paranoia and possibly psychosis for regular, heavy GHB users, which can last many days – similar to the symptoms and signs of alcohol withdrawal. A rapid deterioration into agitated delirium may occur, especially in more frequent high-dose-dependent users. Withdrawal may be treated with benzodiazepines and treatment may be prolonged and require admission to an intensive care unit.

Driving

GHB and GBL can significantly affect driving ability for several hours. Erratic driving may draw attention and drivers have often been found slumped over the steering wheel. Observed effects will be similar to alcohol intoxication and may include dilated pupils, confusion, incoordination, slurred speech and drowsiness, with possible drifting in and out of consciousness after a high dosage. Poor performance on field impairment tests may be expected but the individual may improve rapidly as the drug effects wear off.

Treatment

Diagnosis of intoxication depends on a history of usage together with consistent symptoms over an appropriate time course. There are no specific treatments, although usual basic life support such as maintenance of airway and prevention of vomit aspiration are important.

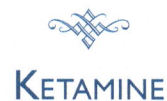

KETAMINE

Principal Drugs and Derivatives

Ketamine, methoxetamine (*N*-ethyl derivative of ketamine).

Common Street Names

Ketamine: special K, vitamin K, K, ket, kit-kat, animal tranquilliser, horse tranquilliser, cat Valium, super acid.
Methoxetamine: m-kat, kmax, MXE, mexxy, legal ketamine.

Mechanism of Action

Dissociative anaesthetic with analgesic and psychedelic properties, central nervous system (CNS) depressants. Ketamine is a non-competitive *N*-methyl-D-aspartate (NMDA) receptor antagonist that interferes with the excitatory amino acids including glutamate and aspartate. The major metabolite of ketamine is norketamine which also possesses some pharmacological activity, although less than the parent drug. Oral effects start within 10–20 min and can last up to 3 h; intravenous effects are experienced within 30 seconds and usually last approximately 30 min; insufflation/snorting effects commence within 5–10 min. The half-life of ketamine is 3–4 h.

Medical Uses (Ketamine)

Ketamine in standard doses is principally used for the induction and maintenance of anaesthesia for surgical procedures. In addition to its

DOI: 10.4324/9781003381730-21

role in anesthesia and analgesia, ketamine has been used in the treatment of asthma, epilepsy, depression, bipolar affective disorders, alcohol and heroin addiction.

There are no medical uses for methoxetamine.

Legal Status

Ketamine is a prescription-only medicine, controlled under the Misuse of Drugs Act 1971, class C in 2006, upgraded to class B in June 2014.

Methoxetamine has been controlled as a class B drug since February 2013.

Presentation and Methods of Administration

Ketamine: sold in liquid form as an anaesthetic, e.g. Ketalar in 10, 50 and 100 mg/mL solutions. Ketamine hydrochloride is found 'on the street' in powder or tablets. It can be taken orally, or by intranasal, intramuscular or intravenous routes.

Methoxetamine: encountered in powder form. Used by nasal insufflation, intravenous and intramuscular injection, sublingually and rectally.

Symptoms and Signs

Acute Intoxication

Physical: cocaine-like rush, vomiting and nausea, slurred speech, nystagmus, ataxia, loss of coordination, pronounced analgesia, numbness, cardiorespiratory stimulant in low doses, with an increase in blood pressure and pulse. Methoxetamine may have greater potency than ketamine and the effects may last longer.

High doses given by rapid intravenous injection may result in the depression of respiration, or apnoea (which is especially dangerous with other CNS depressants), hypertension, tachycardia and neurological toxicity.

Rarely, depression of the laryngeal reflexes predisposes to aspiration and airway obstruction from inhalation of gastric contents.

Psychological: euphoria, psychological dissociation with hallucinations, anxiety, 'out-of-body' experiences (the 'K-hole').

Chronic

Little information is available, but there may be interference with memory, learning and attention. The user may experience flashbacks. There is no physical dependence or withdrawal. Chronic use can lead to significant bladder damage with signs such as ulcers and fibrosis; pain, urinary incontinence and bleeding. It may be necessary to remove the bladder. Methoxetamine was marketed as a 'bladder-safe' version of ketamine but it too has been found to be associated with bladder problems.

Driving

Ketamine may impair driving ability for a few hours and can produce distorted perceptions of space and time, decreased awareness of surroundings, an increase in reaction times and blurred vision. White powder around the nose is a common finding for drivers who have recently used ketamine. Besides driving impairments, recorded psychomotor impairments of the drivers have included dilated pupils, missing or delayed pupil reactions, slurred or decelerated speech, delayed reaction, lack of concentration, vertigo or agitation. Methoxetamine would be expected to act similarly although there have been no controlled driving studies for either drug.

Treatment

After non-medical oral or nasal use all that may be required is rest in a quiet, darkened room.

High doses: intensive observation may be required with mechanical support of respiration. Benzodiazepines may assist treatment of associated anxiety.

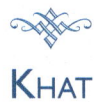

KHAT

Principal Drugs and Derivatives

Khat is an alkaloid (cathinone) derived from the leaves of the khat (qat) shrub – *Catha edulis*. It originates from the Middle East and East Africa. It is structurally similar to amphetamine. Many of the new amphetamine-like synthetic drugs are based on the cathinone chemical structure and are known as synthetic cathinones.

Cathinone is broken down to cathine (norephedrine) and norpseudo-ephedrine. Norephedrine and norpseudoephedrine are the main urinary metabolites, but with some unchanged cathinone also excreted. Use may be detected in urine within 50 min of ingestion – most is excreted by 24 h, but peak plasma levels occur 1–2 h after ingestion. The half-life is 3–6 h.

Manufacture

Cultivated.

Common Street Names

Khat, qat, chat, catha, qaadka, Abyssinian Tea, miraa

Mechanism of Action

Central nervous system stimulant although much milder than amphetamine.

DOI: 10.4324/9781003381730-22

Medical Uses

None.

Legal Status

Cathine and cathinone are class C drugs under schedule 2 of the Misuse of Drugs Act 1971. Khat itself also became a class C controlled drug in the UK in June 2014.

Presentation and methods of administration

Fresh leaves or stalks of the *Catha edulis* plant are chewed (Figure 11). Typically 100–200g of material may be chewed over 3–4 h. It may be drunk as an infusion of leaves (Abyssinian tea).

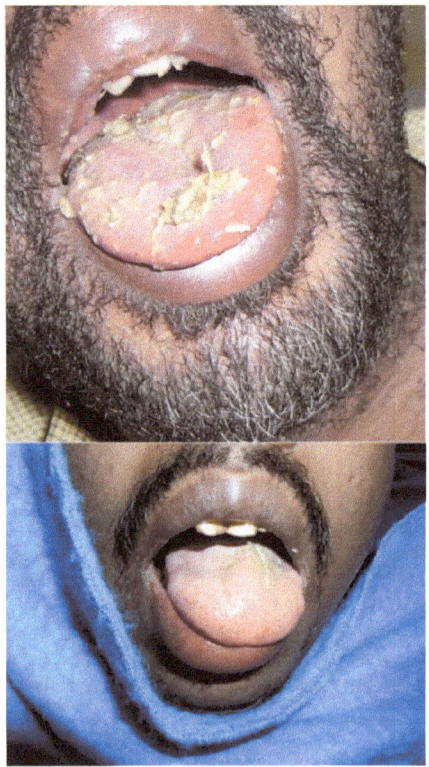

Figure 20.1 *Green discoloration and debris on tongue from chewing khat.*
Source: JJ Payne-James.

Symptoms and Signs

Acute Intoxication

Physical: excitable and talkative, anorexia, tachycardia, insomnia, restlessness, dilated pupils reacting slowly to light, hypertension, palpitations, tremor, flushing lasting for up to 3 h. Poor balance. Impotence may be experienced. The mouth and tongue may become inflamed and painful. The tongue may appear green. Gastritis may be present.
Psychological: sense of wellbeing, irritability, euphoria, excitability, agitation, hyperactivity, hypo-/hypermania or lack of concentration, and can stave off hunger.

General/Chronic

Long-term use may cause bruxism and a personality change. Psychosis (with visual and auditory hallucinations), although rare, has been reported in predisposed individuals. Paranoid delusions may occur. There may be an increased incidence of peptic ulceration. Khat chewing is a risk factor for increased cerebral haemorrhage, cardiomyopathy and myocardial infarction. Khat is associated with several oral and dental conditions, including keratotic white lesions, mucosal pigmentation, periodontal disease, tooth loss, plasma cell stomatitis, and xerostomia.

There appears to be little physical dependence but there may be limited psychological dependence, with withdrawal causing some depression and lethargy.

Cessation/Withdrawal

Long-term users may experience tremor, lassitude and depression on withdrawal.

Driving

Inattention, impaired judgement and coordination may occur; although khat is reported to produce only limited impairment it may cause drowsiness and apathy later. Green and/or brown-coated tongue and teeth may be present. Drivers have been reported to chew khat to stay awake and improve attention.

Treatment

Intoxication: no specific treatment necessary.

General/chronic: no specific treatment required.

Withdrawal: if withdrawal effects are observed, psychological support and counselling may be required.

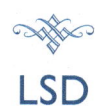

LSD

Principal Drugs and Derivatives

LSD is a semi-synthetic hallucinogen derived from the alkaloid lysergic acid: D-lysergic acid diethylamide, lysergide or LSD-25. Lysergic acid is found in ergot, a fungus which grows on grains such as rye. LSD was first synthesised from lysergic acid in 1938 in Switzerland. 1-Propanoyl-LSD (1P-LSD) is a novel psychoactive substance which is a prodrug of LSD.

Manufacture

Laboratory/factory production.

Common Street Names

Acid, tabs, dots, the cube, microdots, pellets, blue star, trips, California sunshine (and also by the names of the designs used in the manufacture of impregnated paper squares e.g. 'smiley').

Mechanism of Action

After oral intake, effects are present within 60 min and last up to 12 h, peaking at about 4 h. It acts on both the central and the autonomic nervous systems. It is metabolised in the liver and kidneys, with faecal excretion. The main site of action is a serotoninergic receptor $5HT_2$. The half-life of lysergide is 3–5 h.

DOI: 10.4324/9781003381730-23

Medical Uses

None. When first discovered attempts were made to find a use, particularly in psychiatric disorders. Recent research has suggested the possibility of use of LSD in low doses as an analgesic.

Legal Status

LSD is a class A controlled drug under schedule 1 of the Misuse of Drugs Act 1971.

Presentation and Methods of Administration

The amount of LSD required for an effect is very small, typically 25–150 micrograms being adequate, although doses as low as 10 micrograms may be associated with "microdosing" of the drug. It may be produced in the form of tablets (microdots), or impregnated on to blotting paper, sugar cubes or gelatine squares (Figure 12).

Symptoms and Signs

Acute Intoxication

Physical: increased blood pressure, pyrexia, headache, dilatation of the pupils, tachycardia. Tremor, flushing, nausea and temporary loss of

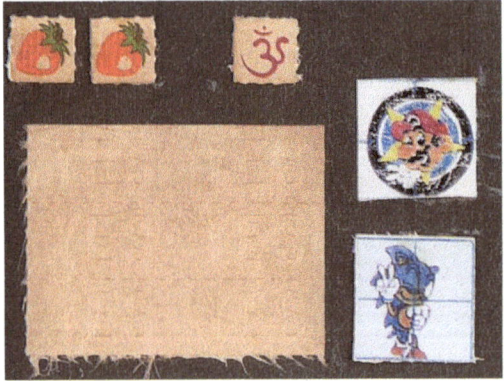

Figure 21.1 *Examples of LSD presentations.*
Source: JJ Payne-James.

appetite may be noted. Some temporary muscular incoordination may be experienced.

Psychological: LSD is known as one of the most potent 'mind-expanding' drugs. Both enjoyable and unpleasant effects (a 'bad trip') may be experienced by users. Its effects vary greatly from individual to individual, and may vary in effect in each individual with repeated use. Effects vary with the individual's current state of mind, personality and environment. Visual hallucinations as well as visual distortion may be experienced. Auditory hallucinations are less common. Perception of time may alter, sometimes passing very slowly and sometimes extremely quickly. The ability to judge distance or speed is reduced. Mood may change acutely from extreme happiness to the depths of depression. Paranoia may be felt, and episodes of violence have been described. As the effects of the drug wear off (over a few hours) periods of normality gradually return.

General/Chronic

Psychological and physical dependence do not occur because tolerance develops rapidly. There may be an increased risk of spontaneous abortion in pregnant women.

Psychological: prolonged psychotic and anxiety reactions occasionally occur.

Flashbacks may occur weeks or months after use.

Cessation/Withdrawal

Withdrawal is not considered a problem, because the nature of the drug generally prevents regular daily use.

Driving

Safe control of a motor vehicle is unlikely given the extreme effects that LSD is capable of producing.

Treatment

Intoxication: supportive treatment while 'trip' is under way.
General/chronic: no specific treatment is required. Disturbing flashbacks have been treated with benzodiazepines.
Withdrawal: no specific treatment is required.

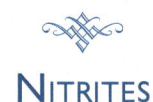

NITRITES

Principal Drugs and Derivatives

Alkyl nitrite, amyl nitrite, butyl nitrite and isobutyl nitrite.

Manufacture

Laboratory/factory production.

Common Street Names

Poppers, bang aroma, liquid gold, locker room, TNT, nitro, ram, rock hard, rush, snapper, stag, stud, thrust.

Mechanism of Action

Alkyl nitrites are volatile liquids (evaporating at normal temperatures) that, following inhalation, deliver a short, sharp 'high', or sense of euphoria and relax smooth muscle, especially in blood vessels and sphincters. The term 'alkyl nitrites' encompasses a group of substances that are chemically similar, with each member of the group differing in the alkyl group it contains (e.g., propyl, butyl). Inhalation of the vapour results in an almost instantaneous but short-lived effect lasting 15–45 min.

Medical Uses

After inhalation nitrites oxidise iron within haemoglobin from the ferrous to the ferric state, forming methaemoglobin. This cannot transport

DOI: 10.4324/9781003381730-24

oxygen around the body and, if sufficient nitrite is ingested, it can lead to methaemoglobinaemia. This can be a useful reaction to utilise after cyanide poisoning because cyanide will very effectively bind to methaemoglobin; consequently administration of amyl nitrite and other methaemoglobin inducers have been used as treatment for cyanide poisoning. Most commonly this group of drugs are used recreationally although arguments have been made that the benefits for receptive anal sex extend beyond making anal sex more pleasurable, to enabling some same-sex couples to engage in sexual intercourse without injury. The use of alkyl nitrites in this context enables sexual functioning for some coupled gay men and thus, has broader benefits to relationship satisfaction and wellbeing.

Legal Status

In the UK, alkyl nitrites have never been controlled via the Misuse of Drugs Act (1971). While use may be associated with harms (including maculopathy and methaemoglobinaemia) the Advisory Council on the Misuse of Drugs recommends that legislation should 'Remove the risk of prosecution under the Psychoactive Substances Act 2016 of those importing, selling or supplying alkyl nitrites to those who wish to use them as an aid to atraumatic sexual intercourse' and notes that '[it] does not recommend that the exemption should be limited to specific alkyl nitrites as there is currently inadequate information about the efficacy and safety of individual products and such a limitation could also cause supply issues in the short to medium term' and the Council 'acknowledges that the exemption would also remove the risk of prosecution under the PSA for those importing, selling or supplying alkyl nitrites for their psychoactive effects'.

Presentation and Methods of Administration

Amyl nitrite is a clear, yellow, volatile, inflammable liquid with a sweet pungent smell.

Commercially it presents as a volatile liquid supplied in glass ampoules historically used recreationally as 'poppers'. (When the ampoule is broken open it 'pops'.) When amyl nitrite is used this way, it is usually inhaled or 'huffed'. Its toxicity is primarily through its oxidative effects and presents as methemoglobinemia. It also acts as a vasodilator.

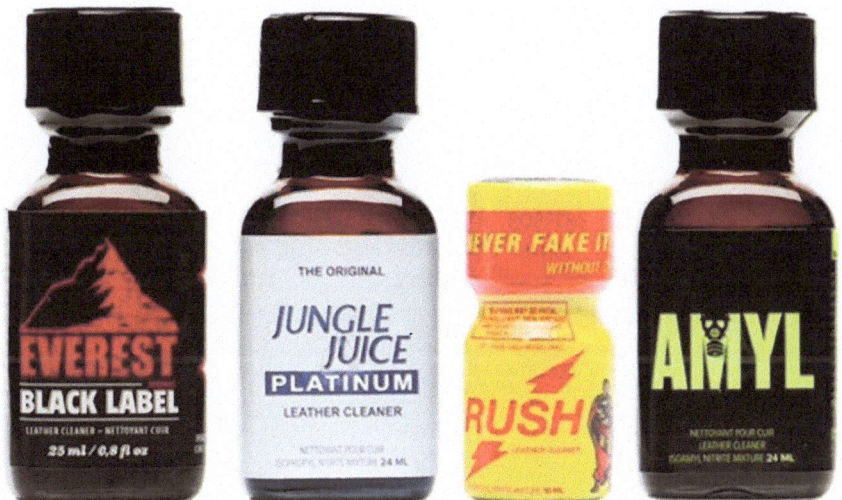

Figure 22.1 *Some examples of the form in which nitrites may be available.*

Nitrites when used as street drugs are usually encountered in small brown glass bottles, frequently sold as room odourisers. The substance can be inhaled directly from the bottle or poured onto a cloth. Poppers are used to enhance sexual performance and relax the anal sphincter. They are also popular among young people to produce rapid euphoriant effects. Typical examples of available nitrite forms are shown in Figure 13.

Symptoms and Signs

Acute Intoxication

Physical: vasodilatation and smooth muscle relaxant, euphoria, cold sweats and hypotension, headache, dizziness, light-headedness, flushed face, weakness, nausea and lacrimation. Severe methaemoglobinaemia (usually >30%) can cause metabolic acidosis, respiratory depression, coma, convulsions and cardiovascular collapse and can be fatal in the absence of treatment. Ventricular fibrillation has been reported.

Chronic

Signs of chronic use are facial dermatitis, an allergic rash and anaemia. Methaemoglobinaemia has been documented. Tolerance does occur but there is no evidence of a physical or psychological dependence.

Driving

The short-lived effects would be incompatible with driving safely when intoxicated.

Treatment

In cases of an overdose remove the person from the exposure and supply oxygen. Serious methaemoglobinaemia may be treated with intravenous methylene blue, e.g. 1.5–2 mg/kg for 5 min together with a litre of intravenous isotonic saline.

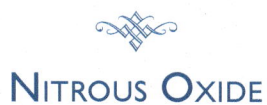

NITROUS OXIDE

Principal Drugs and Derivatives

Nitrous oxide (N2O).

Manufacture

Laboratory/factory production.

Common Street Names

Hippy crack, laughing gas, nangs, N2O, sweet air, whippets, whippits.

Mechanism of Action

Once nitrous oxide is inhaled, the gas enters the blood stream through the lungs and travels to the brain, where it triggers the release of the body's natural opioids, endorphins and dopamine. The anaesthetic effect of nitrous oxide is achieved by temporarily stabilising neuron activity in the brain.

Medical Uses

There is a wide range of legal uses of nitrous oxide, for example pain relief in medical settings, including dentistry. Globally nitrous oxide is the most common inhaled anaesthetic in the medical profession, always administered as a 50/50 blend of nitrous oxide and pure oxygen. In the

DOI: 10.4324/9781003381730-25

non-medical setting it is also used legitimately in industry, for manufacturing and technical processes, such as food packaging, but also in catering, as a whipped cream propellant. Hobbyists also use it in activities such as motorsport drag racing and model rocketry. It is widely available. All sizes of nitrous oxide canisters are illegal if the supplier or owner does not have a legitimate use.

Legal Status

Prior to 8 November 2023, nitrous oxide was subject to the Psychoactive Substances Act 2016. From 8 November 2023 if it is, or is likely to be, wrongfully inhaled, it is classified as a class C drug under the Misuse of Drugs Act 1971. If a person is found in possession of nitrous oxide and intends to wrongfully inhale the substance and/or in the cases of importation, exportation, production and supply, knows or is reckless as to whether it is likely that another person will wrongfully inhale it, they will be committing an offence.

Presentation and Methods of Administration

Nitrous oxide is a colourless non-flammable gas with a pleasant, faintly sweet odour and taste. The most popular method is to 'inhale' the substance from balloons. The balloons themselves are filled with 'nitrous oxide' which is generally being sold in small canisters. Larger compressed canisters may also be available. When used to fill balloons the freezing temperature of the canister pressed against skin can cause frostbite (cold-contact burn) injury.

Symptoms and Signs

Acute Intoxication

Physical: it induces euphoria, relaxation, and hallucinogenic states when inhaled. Acute adverse effects include hypoxia-related seizures and fatality. Inhalation of nitrous oxide has caused pneumothorax, pneumomediastinum, and pneumopericardium.

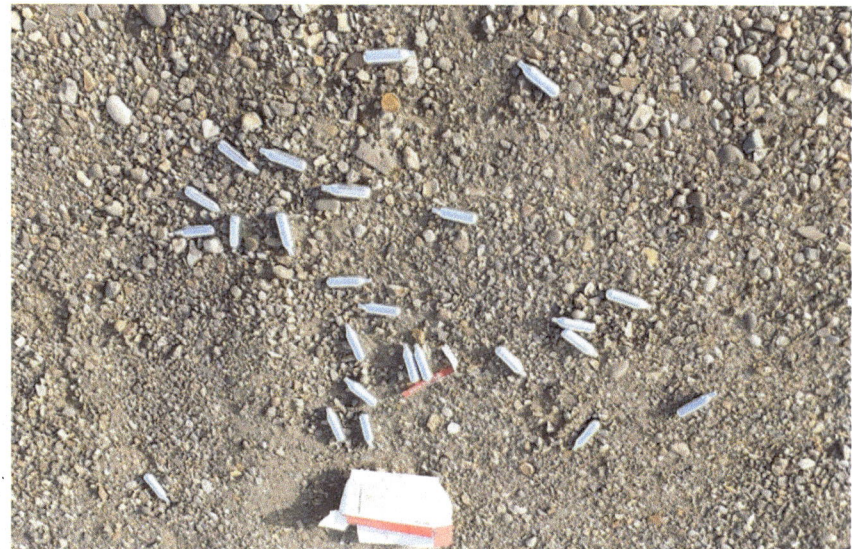

Figure 23.1 *(a) Discarded small volume canisters in a public park.*

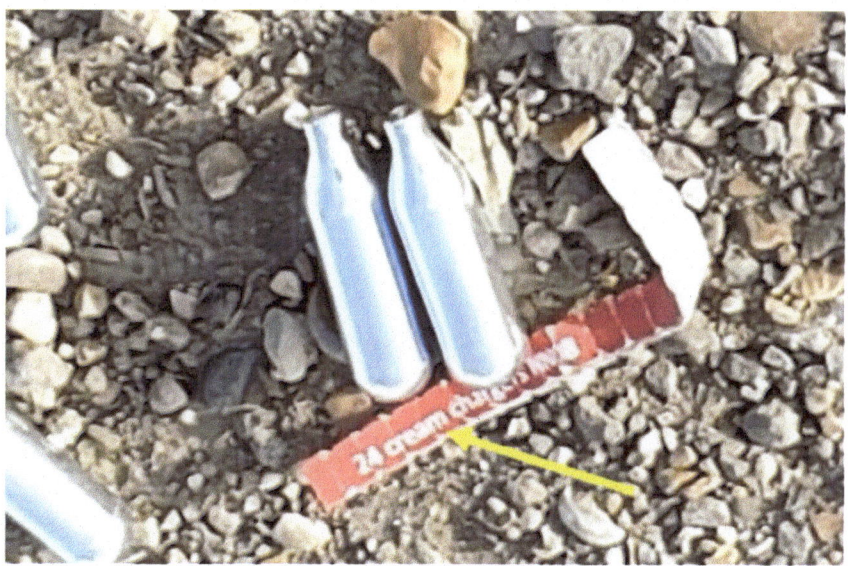

Figure 23.1 *(b) A close-up shows that these canisters originated from chargers from a commercial whipped cream dispenser.*

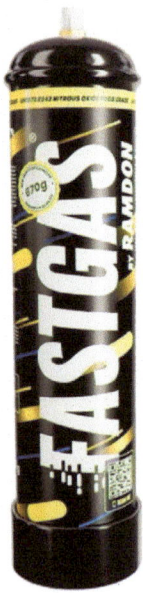

Figure 23.1 *(c) Large volume nitrous oxide canister.*

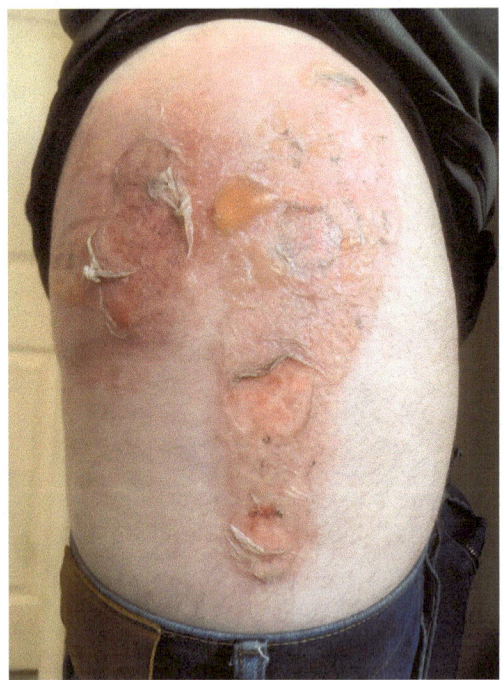

Figure 23.1 *(d) Frostbite injury with a the appearance of a partial thickness cold-contact burn caused from contact with a freezing larger canister used for filling balloons. Source: Figures 14(a-d) JJ Payne-James.*

Chronic

Excessive use can lead to long-term neurological damage. Symptoms include distal paraesthesia, predominantly in the feet but also the hands; unsteadiness on walking; weakness; L'hermitte's phenomenon; bladder or bowel urgency or incontinence; impotence or other sexual dysfunction; segmental myoclonus; mental health issues. Heavy regular use of nitrous oxide can lead to deficiency of vitamin B12 and to a form of anaemia. There have also been cases of nitrous oxide-induced subacute combined degeneration of the cord (N2O-SACD), a pattern of myeloneuropathy usually associated with severe vitamin B12 deficiency. This can cause serious and permanent disability in young people but, if recognised early, may be effectively treated. Severe B12 deficiency can lead to serious nerve damage, causing tingling and numbness in the fingers and toes. This can be very painful and make walking difficult. It can even lead to paralysis, and the damage may be permanent.

Driving

The short-lived effects would be incompatible with driving safely when intoxicated.

Treatment

Ceasing use is critical and patients must be warned that treatment will not work if they continue to use N2O. B12 supplements are required under neurological supervision and may be required for prolonged periods. This regimen is similar to that for traditional SACD. Return to normal function may not ensue. However, relapse following return to N2O use is relatively common, and so patients should be encouraged to contact their local drug and alcohol service to support their abstinence.

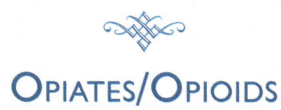

Opiates/Opioids

Principal Drugs

Opiate drugs are derived from the opium plant and include heroin, morphine, codeine and thebaine. Opioids are analogues to these plant-based drugs but are synthetic, (e.g. methadone, tramadol, fentanyls and nitazenes) or semi-synthetic (e.g. buprenorphine).

Medicinal Drugs

Morphine (MST Continus, Oramorph, Cyclimorph) is a strong analgesic prescribed to treat severe pain and is often used in palliative care.

Diamorphine is a strong analgesic prescribed to treat severe pain in an hospital environment only.

Codeine and dihydrocodeine (DHC, DF118) are analgesics used to treat mild to moderate pain, with codeine also being used as a cough suppressant and to treat diarrhoea. Both also occur in combination with other drugs e.g. paracetamol in Co-codamol and Co-dydramol.

Oxycodone (Oxycontin, Oxynorm, Percocet) is an analgesic used to treat moderate to severe pain and may also be used in palliative care.

Methadone hydrochloride (Physeptone) is a synthetic opioid analgesic used widely as a treatment of opioid dependence and occasionally for severe pain.

Buprenorphine (Subutex, Temgesic) is an opioid receptor partial agonist/antagonist and is used in the treatment of opiate dependence.

Suboxone is a combination of buprenorphine and naloxone (as 2 mg/0.5mg or 8 mg/2mg), licensed as a substitution treatment for

DOI: 10.4324/9781003381730-26

opioid dependence. When administered by dissolution under the tongue, as prescribed, very little naloxone reaches the bloodstream because of first-pass metabolism. However, when administered intravenously to opioid-dependent individuals, the naloxone produces marked opioid antagonist effects and causes opioid withdrawal. This acts as a deterrent to intravenous use.

Buprenorphine is also available as an oral lyophilisate (Espranor) and a prolonged release injectable buprenorphine (Buvidal) – given weekly or monthly (various doses).

Tramadol (Zamadol, Zydol) is a mixed-action drug with analgesic effects produced by a combination of weak opioid action and a noradrenergic and serotonin mechanism. It is used to treat moderate to severe pain but is recognised to be used inappropriately.

Fentanyl is a strong analgesic normally used as a patch applied to the skin for transdermal drug transfer to treat chronic intractable pain but recommended for use only in opioid tolerant patients.

Dextromoramide was previously used to treat severe pain but has been withdrawn from use in many countries due to safety concerns.

Dextropropoxyphene, when combined with paracetamol (Co-proxamol), was also used to treat moderate to severe pain but has been withdrawn from use in several countries due to safety concerns.

Pentazocine (Fortran) is used rarely to treat moderate to severe pain.

Dipipanone, with cyclizine (Diconal), is used to treat moderate to severe pain although is now only available in the non-proprietary form in the UK.

Illicit Drugs

A number of synthetic opioids have appeared in the last 10 years or so including AH-7921 and MT-45.

More concerning is the proliferation of fentanyl-related drugs and, more recently, a group of drugs known as nitazenes (2-benzyl benzimidazole compounds) and also brorphine (piperidine benzimidazolone) and related drugs.

Fentanyls include carfentanil, acetylfentanyl, acrylfentanl, butyrfentanyl, 4-fluoroisobutyrfentanyl, cyclopropylfentanyl, methoxyacetylfentanyl, ocfentanil, parafluorofentanyl and furanylfentanyl.

Examples of the nitazene group of drugs which have been encountered include etonitazene, isotonitazene, metonitazene and protonitazene.

Common Street Names

Heroin: skag, smack, gear, shit.
Methadone: amps, linctus, jungle juice.
Buprenorphine: subbies, bupe, temmies.
Oxycodone: oxy, hillbilly heroin.
Dipipanone: dikes.
Fentanyl: china girl, great bear, tango & cash, murder 8.
Nitazenes: iso, tony.

Mechanism of Action

Opiates and opioids are analgesics that depress the central nervous system (CNS) through suppression of noradrenaline; when withdrawal occurs there is a rebound release of noradrenaline. They can be categorised by the specific receptor with which the drug interacts and whether the interaction is agonistic, antagonistic or mixed. Pure agonists include morphine and methadone, pure antagonists include naloxone and naltrexone, mixed agonists/antagonists include pentazocine.

Medical Uses

Uses of opiates and opioids include for pain relief, as cough suppressants and anti-diarrhoeal agents, and for treatment of opiate dependence (methadone and buprenorphine).

Naloxone is used to treat opiate overdose. Naltrexone can be used to prevent relapse in prior opiate-dependent patients and can be formulated with opiate drugs (e.g. buprenorphine) to dissuade excessive dosage being taken.

Legal Status

They are prescription-only medicines, controlled under the Misuse of Drugs Act 1971. It is illegal to possess them without a prescription. Morphine, opium, methadone, dipipanone, dextromoramide, oxycodone, fentanyls, pethidine, AH-7921 and MT-45 are in class A of the Act, dihydrocodeine, codeine and pentazocine in class B, and dextropropoxyphene, tramadol and buprenorphine in class C. In December 2023 the UK's ACMD recommended that nitazenes and brorphine be included within class A of the Act.

Presentation and Methods of Administration

Tablets, linctus, injectable liquid if manufactured; illicit powders.

Heroin can be smoked, sniffed or injected (as 'brown', i.e. heroin base powder, heroin will need to be dissolved in an acid, usually citric or ascorbic acid, before intravenous injection; Figure 15); most other preparations can be injected or taken orally. Intravenous injection of heroin (mainlining) results in an almost instantaneous effect or 'rush', whereas injection into muscle, or subcutaneously (skin popping), gives a slower and less intense effect. Sniffing will also result in a less intense effect, but the effects of smoking ('chasing the dragon') are almost as quick as an intravenous injection.

Fentanyl and related drugs can be encountered in many forms including powders, liquids and in counterfeit tablets, particularly those purporting to contain oxycodone. Such compounds are far more potent than morphine, e.g. carfentanil is 10,000 times more potent, with consequent adverse outcomes more likely following use of such drugs. Compounding this, users will frequently have no idea of the strength of the preparation being taken, making overdose a realistic possibility. Proliferation of fentanyl and related drugs has led to an opioid epidemic in North America with many 100,000s of deaths.

Nitazenes are typically encountered as yellow, brown or off-white powders, liquids and nasal sprays but also as counterfeit tablets, again particularly those purporting to contain oxycodone. Potency is again an issue with such compounds being 100 to 500 times more potent than morphine.

Fentanyl and related drugs, and nitazenes, may sometimes be added to heroin powders, massively increasing the overall potency and the subsequent risk of overdosage with severe respiratory depression and death being possible outcomes. They may also be combined with benzodiazepine drugs ('benzo-dope').

Medicinal preparations include the following:

- Morphine: tablets and capsules including sustained release 5, 10, 15, 30, 60, 100 and 200 mg; oral solutions, injection ampoules (1 mg/mL, 10 mg/mL), suppositories. Variable onset and duration of effects depending on formulation taken.
- Diamorphine

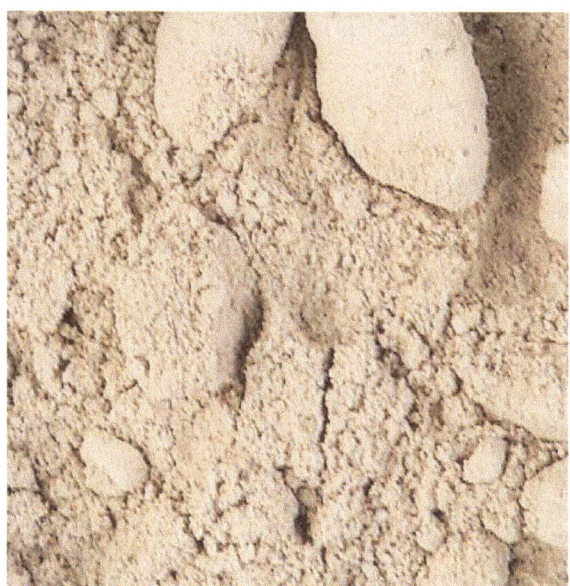

Figure 24.1 *Appearance of powdered heroin ('brown').*
Source: JJ Payne-James.

- Codeine
- Dihydrocodeine
- Methadone: tablets containing methadone hydrochloride 5 mg; methadone mixture (1 mg/mL), a viscous syrupy liquid, which can be colourless or coloured, containing methadone hydrochloride. A blue hyperconcentrated solution may also be available at 10 mg/mL; a weaker form, methadone linctus, is available at a strength of 2 mg/5 mL; methadone injection clear, colourless liquid in ampoules of 1 mL, 2 mL, 3.5 mL and 5 mL containing methadone hydrochloride BP 10 mg/mL.
- Oxycodone: tablets at strengths of 5, 10, 20, 40 or 80 mg; oral solutions 5 mg/5 mL, 10 mg/mL and injection ampoules.
- Buprenorphine: tablets 200 µg or 400 mg, injection ampoules 300 mg, and patches 5, 10 or 20 mg/h for 7 days. It is a partial agonist with a long duration of action. It is an effective analgesic and can be taken sublingually or by injection.
- Fentanyl: patch 12 or 25 µg per hour (replaced after 72 hours); buccal and sublingual tablets 100, 200, 300, 400, 600, 800 µg.
- Tramadol: tablets and capsules 50 mg; sustained release 50 or 100mg.

Symptoms and Signs

Acute Intoxication

Physical: pinpoint (constricted) pupils, depression of the heart rate and respiration, suppression of the cough reflex, constipation, drowsiness and sleep. Nausea and vomiting can occur. High doses can result in respiratory arrest, unconsciousness and death.

Complications may arise due to impurities injected with illicit heroin (including anthrax). Media reports of deaths due to 'contaminated' heroin are normally incorrect and fatality has usually been caused by a batch of heroin with higher than normal purity reaching the end-user or due to other drugs being added such as a fentanyl or nitazene-type drug. Smoking heroin is a safer mode of use than injection.

Psychological: opioids reduce anxiety, produce pain relief and euphoria, a feeling of contentment and an inability to concentrate. There is little interference with mental or physical functioning. The general depressant effects of opioids may be enhanced by other agents with CNS depressant activity such as alcohol, benzodiazepines, tricyclic antidepressants and phenothiazines. Heroin and/or methadone and alcohol together are a particularly dangerous combination.

Chronic

Tolerance and physical and psychological dependence occur and few will be unaware of the opioid crisis of addiction and deaths particularly in the USA and other associated harms of the opioid epidemic. However, tolerance does not develop to all the effects of opiates because increasing doses have to be taken to achieve the same analgesic or euphoric effect, although pupillary constriction will usually remain constant. Cross-tolerance does occur between the various opiates. If drug administration is stopped, e.g. by a period of imprisonment, tolerance will be lost and there is a risk that, if the previous dose is taken, fatal intoxication can occur. The severity of physical dependence depends on the particular opiate used, the dose and the duration of administration. Psychological dependence on opiates is severe and persists after the physical withdrawal syndrome has passed. There is therefore a high relapse rate of opiate dependence.

Amenorrhoea, loss of libido and chronic constipation occur. Women generally remain fertile despite the menstrual irregularity. Opiate use during pregnancy may result in 'small-for-dates' babies who themselves may suffer severe withdrawal syndrome after birth.

Withdrawal

The onset, peak and duration of symptoms of the withdrawal syndrome will depend on which opiate is misused, e.g. heroin withdrawal will have an earlier onset, and be of shorter duration and greater intensity when compared with methadone. The expectation of withdrawal and psychological factors are also important. Effects start within 8–24 h after the last dose and may last up to 10 days. After chronic administration of buprenorphine the onset of the withdrawal syndrome is delayed, with only mild signs from 3–10 days.

Symptoms: yawning, feelings of hot and cold, anorexia, abdominal cramps, nausea, vomiting, diarrhoea, tremor, insomnia, generalised aches and weakness.

Signs: dilated pupils, gooseflesh, flushing, sweating, rhinorrhoea or lacrimation, tachycardia (a pulse rate of 10 beats/min over the baseline or >90 beats/min if no history of tachycardia), hypertension (systolic blood pressure ≥10 mm Hg above baseline or >160/96 in non-hypertensive patients), increased bowel sounds and restlessness.

An opiate withdrawal scale may be useful in certain settings to determine the degree of withdrawal and assess response to therapy (see Appendix C).

Opiate withdrawal during pregnancy can result in fetal death and premature labour. Therefore maintenance therapy with substitute opioids is preferred.

Driving

All opioid drugs are capable of producing effects such as drowsiness, lack of concentration, lack of coordination and slowed reaction times, resulting in poor performance on tasks requiring divided attention, including driving. The effects on any particular individual's driving ability will depend on factors such as how much is taken, the method of administration and the person's tolerance to the drug.

Some of the longer-acting drugs, such as methadone, may not adversely affect driving ability once a person is maintained on a regular daily dose. Codeine, dihydrocodeine, oxycodone and tramadol are only likely to produce significant adverse effects if taken in excessive dosage. Use of heroin or other illicit opiates/opioids is not compatible with safe driving.

Treatment

Overdose: naloxone is a specific opioid antagonist and is given in a dose of 0.4 mg, which can be repeated at intervals of 2–3 min up to a maximum of 10 mg. If there is no effect then the diagnosis of opiate overdose should be reconsidered. Naloxone has a short half-life, so observation in hospital is required after treatment. Naloxone can be given intravenously or intramuscularly (it may be difficult to establish intravenous access) where it is has a longer duration of action.

Emergency medicine advice suggests supplemental oxygen or bag-valve-mask ventilation where RR < 10/minute or SpO2 < 92% (on air).

Naloxone is now available as Nyxoid, a single-dose nasal spray containing 1.8 mg of naloxone.

Naloxone administration is not without risk in the opiate-dependent individual and it may precipitate the opiate withdrawal syndrome, which is distressing but short-lived. Rarely hypertension, pulmonary oedema and cardiac dysrhythmias may occur.

Naltrexone is a specific opioid antagonist in tablet form and is used as an adjunctive therapy in the maintenance of detoxified former opioid-dependent patients.

Withdrawal

The drugs in Table 24.1 can be used in the symptomatic treatment of opiate withdrawal.

Substitution for heroin can be used with a variety of drugs – methadone, buprenorphine, codeine or dihydrocodeine are examples.

If there is doubt about the daily dose of methadone, this can be divided and the condition of the patient reviewed after a proportion has been administered.

Naltrexone is a pure opiate antagonist with a long half-life. It can be taken orally and blocks the effects of opiates for 72 h, so it can be administered three times a week.

It should not be given to an individual who is still dependent on opiates until 7–10 days after the last ingestion of opiates, otherwise it will precipitate a withdrawal reaction that will be protracted because of naltrexone's long duration of action.

TABLE 24.1 Symptomatic Treatment Of Opiate Withdrawal

Symptom	Drug	Administration
Vomiting	Metoclopramide	10mg three times daily. Not known to be harmful in pregnancy. Action antagonised by opioid analgesics. Caution, especially in young adults (15-19 yrs), extrapyramidal effects commonly occur.
	Buccal prochlorperazine	3 or 6mg (one or two 3mg tablets) absorbed from buccal cavity twice daily. Useful if unable to retain oral medication.
Abdominal cramps	Mebeverine hydrochloride	135-150mg three times daily, preferably 20 minutes before meals. Antispasmodic, not known to be harmful in pregnancy.
	Hyoscine butylbromide	10-20mg four times daily Smooth muscle relaxant Advised to avoid in pregnancy
Diarrhoea	Loperamide	Loperamide 4mg initially followed by one after each loose stool; maximum 16mg daily. An opiate receptor agonist which acts on the gut to reduce peristalsis, increase intestinal transit time and increase tone of the anal sphincter.
Minor aches and pains	Paracetamol	Paracetamol 500mg x 2 up to four times a day (maximum eight per day).
	NSAID such as ibuprofen	Ibuprofen 200-400mg three to four times daily (max 2.4g daily. Avoid in pregnancy especially third trimester.

Faculty of Forensic and Legal Medicine and Royal College of Psychiatrists, 2020. *Detainees with Substance Use Disorders in Police Custody Guidelines for Clinical Management*, fifth edition. Report of a Medical Working Group. Council report CR227, London: Royal College of Psychiatrists. Available from: www.fflm.ac.uk (accessed 28 Jan 2024).

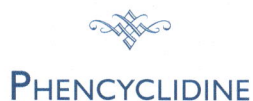

PHENCYCLIDINE

Principal Drugs and Derivatives

Phencyclidine (PCP) or phencyclidine hydrochloride or phenylcyclo-hexyl piperidine or 1-[1-phenylcyclohexyl]-piperidine. First developed as an anaesthetic agent in 1959.

Manufacture

Laboratory/factory production; may be diverted from veterinary sources.

Common Street Names

Angel dust, dust, crystal, rocket fuel, peace pill, crystal joints, sawgrass, zoom, the sheets, and elephant tranquilizer. The drug may be mixed with other drugs including crack cocaine (known as 'space base') and cannabis (crystal supergrass, love-boat, killer weed).

Mechanism of Action

Dependent on dosage, it may act as a dissociative anaesthetic, a stimulant, depressant or hallucinogen because it has mixed neurological effects. The drug can cause dissociative effects.

Effects are observed within 30 min if taken orally, but within 5 min if smoked or injected. Acute effects will last for up to 6 h, with a return to normality within 24 h. The half-life is 21 h.

DOI: 10.4324/9781003381730-27

Medical Uses

Originally an anaesthetic drug for human and veterinary use. It has not been used in the medical setting for several decades, and was withdrawn in 1965 because of dissociative hallucinogenic effects that were often disturbing and sometimes severe and prolonged.

Legal Status

Phencyclidine is classified as class A under the Misuse of Drugs Act 1971 and schedule 2 under the Misuse of Drugs Regulations 2001.

Presentation and Methods of Administration

PCP is a crystalline white powder, readily soluble in water or alcohol. It can be ingested orally, injected intravenously, inhaled, or smoked. It may be encountered as a liquid, and in this form can be smoked, taken orally or intranasally, or injected intravenously.

Symptoms and Signs

Acute Intoxication

Physical: at lower to moderate doses (<10 mg) there may be loss of coordination, slurred speech, skin flushing, increased muscle tone, numbness of the limbs and sweating, tachycardia, tachypnoea and hypertension. The user may show a fixed blank stare and repetitive incoherent speech. At higher doses (>10 mg) blood pressure, pulse and respiratory rate may all decrease. Vertical nystagmus, visual disturbance, excessive salivation and nausea may be experienced. The anaesthetic properties of PCP may render the individual less sensitive to pain, allowing injuries to go unnoticed. Rhabdomyolysis, hypoglycemia, seizures, hypertensive crisis, coma, respiratory arrest and death are some of the complications that can arise with PCP use.

Psychological: lower doses may cause irritability, euphoria or anxiety and, as doses increase, disturbances of body image, aggression and paranoia can be experienced. Auditory hallucinations will be observed with higher doses and episodes of bizarre behaviour are common. Paranoid delusions become increased and the individual may react to perceived threats with frightening physical violence.

General/Chronic

Physical: no physical dependence occurs.

Psychological: there is some evidence that psychological dependence develops. Memory may be affected. Drug-induced psychosis after use of PCP may last up to several weeks, particularly in those with a history of psychiatric disorders such as schizophrenia. Tolerance may develop and craving for the drug may occur.

Cessation/Withdrawal

Depression and social withdrawal are common sequelae of chronic PCP misuse. There may be a mild abstinence syndrome with depression and disorientation.

Driving

PCP has been shown to produce significant disorientation, drowsiness, lack of attention and coordination, slowed reaction time and impaired perception of space. These effects may last in excess of 12 h after use. All are likely to be incompatible with driving a motor vehicle but no known studies. Ketamine (a phencyclidine derivative) has been shown to affect driving ability.

Treatment

Intoxication: acidification of the urine may reduce the drug half-life by accelerating excretion. Haloperidol has been used and evaluated, orally, intramuscularly and intravenously.

General/chronic: no specific treatment.

Withdrawal: standard treatment(s) for depressive episodes when clinically indicated.

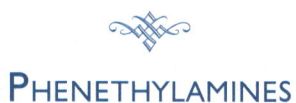

PHENETHYLAMINES

Principal Drugs and Derivatives

A huge range of compounds falls within this very broad category of drugs of substituted phenylethylamines. Within the category the so-called '2C' group comprises phenethylamines with methoxy groups on the 2 and 5 positions of the benzene ring, including:

- 2-CB (4-bromo-2,5-dimethoxyphenethylamine) (one of the most commonly used)
- 2-CE (2,5-dimethoxy-4-ethylphenethylamine)
- 2-CI (2,5-dimethoxy-4-iodophenethylamine)
- 25B-NBOMe (4-bromo-2,5-dimethoxy-N-(2-methoxyphenyl) phenethylamine)
- 25I-NBOMe (4-iodo-2,5-dimethoxy-N-(2-methoxyphenyl) phenethylamine)
- 25C-NBOMe (4-chloro-2,5-dimethoxy-N-(2-methoxyphenyl) phenethylamine)
- DOI (2,5-dimethoxy-4-iodo-amphetamine)
- DOM (2,5-dimethoxy-4-methylamphetamine).

Other structurally related drugs include 2CB-FLY (2-(8-bromo-2,3,6,7-tetrahydrofuro [2,3-f][1]benzofuran-4-yl)ethanamine), Bromodragonfly (1-(4-bromofuro[2,3-f] benzofuran-8-yl)propan-2-amine) and mescaline (3,4,5-trimethoxyphenethylamine).

DOI: 10.4324/9781003381730-28

Manufacture

Illicit laboratories; mescaline occurs naturally in the peyote cactus (*Lophophora williamsii*), native to southern North America and the San Pedro cactus (*Echinopsis pachanoi*), native to South America, and a few other plant species.

Common Street Names

Nexus, bromo, N-bomb, Europa, CBs, bomb-25, smiley paper.

Mechanism of Action

These act as central nervous system stimulants but often with powerful hallucinogenic effects. To a lesser extent, they act as neurotransmitters in the human central nervous system. There is no mechanism of action or biological target that is common to all compounds. They are absorbed by the gastrointestinal tract and may have an effect within 20 min of ingestion. Some compounds have delayed action, and some have a very steep dose–response curve, so there can be large differences in effects and duration even with a small variation in dosage. Active dosages for many of these drugs are very low with as little as 0.1 mg being required for the 'N-bomb' drugs. Others may require up to 5 mg although a typical dose of 2C-B is 10–25 mg. Large dosages of some drugs may produce effects lasting more than 24 h. Half-lives for most of these drugs have not been established.

Medical Uses

None.

Legal Status

All classified as class A under the Misuse of Drugs Act 1971 and schedule 1 under the Misuse of Drugs Regulations 2001.

Presentation and Methods of Administration

Taken orally or by snorting but can be taken sublingually or via injection. Usually available in form of pills, capsules and tablets, but compounds can be sold in powder form, while oral doses (on a slip of blotter paper) are usually available for 'D substances'. Ingestion is the most common route of administration of phenethylamines.

Symptoms and Signs

Acute Intoxication

Physical: effects are very varied; can include poor coordination; mood elevation; giggling/smiling; muscle spasms; tremors; bruxism; tachycardia; tachypnoea; wakefulness; self-confidence, talkativeness and agitation. Produces adrenaline-like effects. Phenethylamines cause headache; hypertension; tachycardia; dry mouth and sweating. Limb ischaemia and fatality can occur.

Psychological: psychedelic effects, sometimes in waves. Higher doses can result in irrational behaviour, confusion, fear, hallucinations, delusions, paranoia and psychosis.

General/Chronic

Unknown. Enduring psychosis has been reported after a single dose.

Driving

All likely to be incompatible with driving a motor vehicle but no known studies.

Treatment

Intoxication: nil – unless complications develop. Then supportive with monitoring of vital signs in hospital setting; intravenous benzodiazepines may be appropriate.

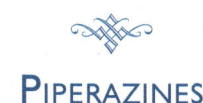

PIPERAZINES

Principal Drugs and Derivatives

1-Benzylpiperazine (BZP), 1-(3-trifluoromethylphenyl) piperazine (TFMPP), 1-(3-chlorophenyl)piperazine (mCPP).

Manufacture

Illicit laboratories; mCPP is a metabolite of trazodone. Do not occur in nature.

Common Street Names

Legal E, legal X, herbal ecstasy, BZPs, party pills, pep pills, social tonics, Jax, A2, benny bear, flying angel, pep X, pep love or nemesis, fast lane, exodus, cosmic kelly, bolts extra strength, blast. MCPP is known as 3CPP, 3Cl-PP or CPP.

Mechanism of Action

They are central nervous system stimulants although they are less potent than amphetamine and MDMA. TFMPP produces fewer stimulant effects than BZP and is associated with increased anxiety; mCPP can produce unpleasant effects and is less desirable to users. TFMPP and mCPP may produce hallucinogenic effects. BZP is believed to cause the release of dopamine and noradrenaline and inhibition of monoamine uptake, causing tachycardia and hypertension. Hallucinogenic effects of BZP at high doses may be due to binding with $5HT_{2a}$ receptors. Piperazines are

DOI: 10.4324/9781003381730-29

absorbed by the gastrointestinal tract and the effects commence within 20 min of ingestion and last for up to 8 h. Dosage range is normally up to 200 mg for BZP, but ≤100 mg for TFMPP. BZP and TFMPP are sometimes encountered together e.g. as a 10:1 mix. The half-life for BZP is reported as 5.5 h.

Medical Uses

A number of piperazine compounds have an anthelmintic action for use in worm infections.

Legal Status

Piperazines are classified class C under the Misuse of Drugs Act 1971.

Presentation and Methods of Administration

Typically powder or tablet form. May be liquids.

Symptoms and Signs

Acute Intoxication

Physical: anxiety, vomiting, sweating, headache and palpitations. They may have behavioral, neuroendocrine, psychostimulatory and hallucinogenic effects. Seizures, respiratory and metabolic acidosis have been reported. Hyperthermia, rhabdomyolysis and renal failure have been documented. Deaths have been reported.
Psychological: difficulties sleeping, mood swings, loss of energy, irritability, confusion. Higher doses can result in unpredictable and serious toxicity including seizures and collapse.

General/Chronic

Unknown.

Driving

A study showed that BZP/TFMPP improved driving performance by improving attention and decreasing weaving of the vehicle. However, the study was stopped early due to the high incidence of severe adverse events including agitation, anxiety, hallucinations, vomiting, insomnia and migraine.

Treatment

Intoxication: nil – unless complications develop. Then treatment is supportive with monitoring of vital signs in a hospital setting; intravenous benzodiazepines may be appropriate.

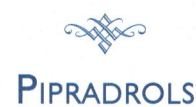

PIPRADROLS

Principal Drugs and Derivatives

Desoxypipradrol, diphenylprolinol, diphenylmethylpyrrolidine.

Common Street Names

D2PM, 2-DPMP; ivory wave; head candy; whack; neuroblast. Have been marketed as being 'not for human consumption' and 'research chemicals'.

Mechanism of Action

Selective catecholamine uptake inhibitors. Central nervous system stimulants increasing dopamine release and also decreasing dopamine reuptake. Absorbed by the gastrointestinal tract with effects commencing within 20 minutes of oral ingestion, with a faster onset if snorted. The effects can be long lasting, up to several days.

Medical Uses

No medical uses. Pipradrol was originally used for the treatment of attention deficit hyperactivity disorder (ADHD), obesity, narcolepsy and depression.

Legal Status

Pipradrol is classified as class C under the Misuse of Drugs Act 1971 and schedule 3 under the Misuse of Drugs Regulations 2001.

DOI: 10.4324/9781003381730-30

Presentation and Methods of Administration

Tablets, capsules or powder. May be taken orally or snorted. The typical dosage is within a range of 10 to 25 mg.

Symptoms and Signs

Acute Intoxication

Physical: tachycardia, hypertension, sweating, bruxism, agitation, rhabdomyolysis. These effects may last several days but generally wear off of their own accord. There is a prolonged psychostimulant action. Neuropsychiatric effects may last up to a week after ingestion. A toxidrome lasting days with tachycardia, tachypnoea, dystonia, rhabdomyolysis, leucocytosis, agitation, hallucinations, insomnia and paranoia have been reported with desoxypipradrol. Deaths have been reported.
Psychological: euphoria, paranoia, psychosis.

General/Chronic

Physical: long-term use. No information available.
Psychological: in addition to the short-term effects continued usage could cause aggression, fatigue, weakness, insomnia, anxiety, depression, psychosis. They have addictive potential.

Cessation/Withdrawal

Cessation can cause anxiety and depression, disturbance of sleep patterns, irritability.

Driving

No published controlled studies but would be expected to produce similar effects to other stimulant drugs for example, increased risk-taking, impatience and driving at high speed. Physical signs may include restlessness, agitation and aggression. Desoxypipradrol has been identified in driving under the influence cases.

Treatment

Intoxication: nil – unless complications develop. Then supportive with monitoring of vital signs in hospital setting. Benzodiazepines may be useful to treat agitation.

General/chronic: as for intoxication.

Withdrawal: psychological support and counselling.

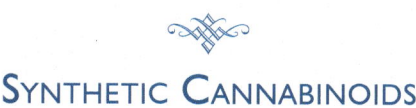

SYNTHETIC CANNABINOIDS

Principal Drugs and Derivatives

JWH-018, JWH-022, JWH-073, JWH-122, JWH-210, HU-210, CP47, AM-694, AM-2201, UR-144, PB-22, RCS-4, URB-597, APINACA, MDMB-4en-PINACA, 5F-ADB and very many others. Several hundred different 'spice' compounds have been identified.

Common Street Names

Spice, spice gold, spice silver, K2, herbal incense, herbal smoking blends, black mamba, potpourri, annihilation, bliss, fake weed, blaze, fake weed, joker.

Manufacture

Synthetic cannabinoids are compounds made in the laboratory to structurally and functionally mimic phytocannabinoids from the cannabis sativa L. plant, including delta-9-tetrahydrocannabinol (THC).

Mechanism of Action

Synthetic cannabinoids are a class of designer drug molecules that bind to the same receptors to which cannabinoids (THC, CBD and many others) in cannabis plants attach. Most of these compounds target the CB1 cannabinoid receptor, producing peripheral and central nervous system effects. There is increasing evidence for parent drugs, and metabolites, binding to CB2 cannabinoid receptors. Many are more potent

DOI: 10.4324/9781003381730-31

than tetrahydrocannabinol (THC) with JWH-018 having 4x, JWH-122 60x and JWH-210 90x the potency of THC. They are abused for their euphoric, energising and disinhibitory effects. There are few studies of the half-life, but it is probably very short, e.g. JWH-018 about 2 h.

Medical Uses

Some have been licenced for the treatments of medication-related nausea. Some may have a role in the treatment of other conditions including neuropathic pain, spasticity-related pain, fibromyalgia, osteoarthritis, and postoperative pain.

Legal Status

The Misuse of Drugs Act 1971 (Amendment) Order 2013 amends the generic definition of controlled synthetic cannabinoid receptor agonists (commonly known as 'synthetic cannabinoids'). They are classified as class B drugs under schedule 2 of the Misuse of Drugs Act 1971. The Psychoactive Substances Act 2016 created a blanket ban on the import, production, supply, and possession (in custodial settings) of all synthetic cannabinoids and novel psychoactive substances in the UK.

Presentation and Methods of Administration

Powdered chemicals, dissolved and sprayed onto paper or dried plant material. They are also available as pure compounds and can be made into a concentrated liquid to be used in vapes. A typical dosage is <10 mg of active constituent, often 1–2 mg.

Symptoms and Signs

Acute Intoxication

Physical: tachycardia, hypertension, hallucinations, nausea and vomiting, chest pain, seizures, somnolence, dilated pupils, respiratory depression, acute kidney injury. Use may lead to the need for hospital attendance with unwanted and/or frightening symptoms including inability to move, dizziness, breathing difficulties, extreme anxiety, paranoia, suicidal thoughts, psychosis.

Hyperpyrexia has been described and acute behavioural disturbance (ABD) may occur. Can alter cerebral blood flow, leading to cerebrovascular complications including ischaemic stroke, subarachnoid hemorrhage, and reversible cerebral vasoconstriction syndrome (RCVS).

Psychological: acute anxiety, psychosis and memory changes.

General/Chronic

Chronic use may be associated with increased risk of long-term cognitive deficits, schizophrenia, and other neuropsychiatric effects. Multiple reports link consumption to various adverse health effects, which is a public health concern.

Physical: Cardiovascular effects include acute cardiac toxicities, hypertension, tachycardia, myocardial infarction, and cardiac arrest. Arrhythmias include sinus bradycardia, second-degree atrioventricular block, ventricular fibrillation, and atrial fibrillation. Acute kidney injury and tubular necrosis has been documented. Liver function derangement and liver failure have been documented.

Psychological: psychoses including episodes of visual and auditory hallucinations, paranoid delusions, anxiety, insomnia and suicidal ideation. Moderate levels of dependence risks.

Cessation/Withdrawal

Particularly after long-term use withdrawal symptoms include: headaches, anxiety, low mood, difficulty concentrating, irritability, restlessness, drug craving, nocturnal nightmares, sweating, tremor and nausea.

Driving

Synthetic cannabinoids appear to impair psychomotor performance in humans, affecting different domains related to safe driving even at low doses.

Treatment

Intoxication: nil – unless complications develop. Then treatment is supportive with monitoring of vital signs in a hospital setting.
General/chronic: as for intoxication.
Withdrawal: psychological support and counselling.

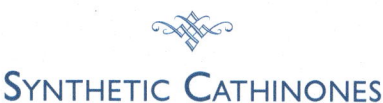

SYNTHETIC CATHINONES

Principal Drugs and Derivatives

Synthetic cathinones, derived from cathinone found in the plant Catha edulis, represent the second largest and most frequently seized group of novel psychoactive substances. They include mephedrone (4-methylmethcathinone), 4-methylethcathinone, methedrone (4-methoxymethcathinone), MDPV (3,4-methylenedioxy-pyrovalerone), methylone (3,4-methylenedioxy-methylcathinone), butylone (methylenedioxy-phenyl-2-methylaminobutanone), flephedrone (4-fluoromethcathinone), naphyrone (naphthylpyrovalerone), methcathinone, buphedrone, bupropion.

Manufacture

Laboratory/factory production.

Common Street Names

Bath salts, legal highs, plant food, NRG-1, NRG-2, MCAT, ivory wave, miaow-miaow, 4-MMC, 4-MEC, MMCAT, 4-FMC, bubbles, rush, stardust, vanilla sky, ocean burst, blizzard, pure ivory. Sellers, buyers and users often have no idea which of these drugs they are providing or using.

Mechanism of Action

These drugs are central nervous system stimulants of varying potency; they also have a psychostimulant action with some effects resembling

DOI: 10.4324/9781003381730-32

MDMA. They are considered as β-keto analogs of amphetamine, sharing pharmacological effects with amphetamine and cocaine. They cause neuroinflammation, dysregulate neurotransmitter systems, and alter monoamine transporters and receptors. They are absorbed by the gastrointestinal tract and effects commence within 20 min of oral ingestion, faster if snorted. The effect is immediate if injected. The effects last 1–4 h, and the compounds are mostly metabolised by the liver. They are heavily metabolised but some drug may be eliminated unchanged in the urine. Half-lives have not been established.

Medical Uses

No medical use.

Legal Status

Cathinone is classified as class C under the Misuse of Drugs Act 1971 and schedule 1 under the Misuse of Drugs Regulations 2001. Cathinone derivatives are classified as class B and schedule 1.

Presentation and Methods of Administration

Tablets, capsules, powder. May be taken orally, sniffed, snorted, smoked or injected.

Typical dosages depend on the specific drug, the route of administration and drug purity e.g. mephedrone dosage may be up to 250 mg if taken orally but 150 mg if snorted; MDPV dosage is much lower being 5 to 20 mg.

Symptoms and Signs

Acute Intoxication

Physical: low-to-moderate doses may produce tachypnoea, tachycardia, hypertension, loss of appetite, dilatation of pupils, brisk reflexes, fine tremor of limbs, agitation, insomnia, nausea, headache, body odour and memory loss. Higher doses will produce dry mouth, pyrexia, sweating, blurring of vision, dizziness, bruxism, flushing or pallor, cardiac dysrhythmias, loss of coordination, hallucinations, delirium, seizures, paranoia or vomiting. These effects may last several hours depending on the drug used and dosage, but generally wear off of their own accord. Deaths have been reported.

Psychological: euphoria, feeling of self-confidence, raised self-esteem, lowered anxiety, increased energy, greater concentration, empathy, openness, increased libido, irritability, restlessness. Higher doses can result in irrational behaviour, confusion, fear, hallucinations, memory loss, delusions, paranoia or psychosis. Acute behavioural disturbance (ABD) and serotonin syndrome have been documented. Psychological dependence has been observed although, as yet, physical dependence is not generally considered to occur. A strong craving to repeat or increase dosage is common.

If injected the user additionally experiences a sensory 'rush' or 'flash' – giving almost immediate sensations of enhanced energy and self-confidence and enhanced sexual enjoyment.

General/Chronic

Longer-term use may require increased dosage levels due to tolerance. Some of these drugs may be used over a period of days until the supply has been exhausted (provoking comparison with cocaine binges), after which the user may be completely exhausted and consequently sleep for several days. Brain-related adverse effects, include encephalopathy, coma and convulsions, and sympathomimetic and hallucinogenic toxidromes. Synthetic cathinone consumption is associated with the risk of developing psychotic symptoms as indicated by the prevalence of hallucinations and/or delusions but evidence of synthetic cathinone-induced psychosis is not clear.

Physical: long-term use. Limited information is currently available because of their only recent increased usage.

Psychological: in addition to the short-term effects, continued usage can cause aggression, insomnia, anxiety, depression and psychosis. They appear to have significant addictive potential.

Cessation/Withdrawal

Users find that cessation can cause anxiety and depression, disturbance of sleep patterns and irritability.

Driving

Some studies have published findings in drivers who have taken synthetic cathinones. Synthetic cathinones would be expected to produce similar effects to other stimulant drugs, e.g. increased risk taking, impatience and driving at high speed. Physical signs may include dilated pupils, restlessness, agitation and aggression.

Treatment

Intoxication: nil – unless complications develop, then supportive with monitoring of vital signs in hospital setting. Benzodiazepines may be useful to treat agitation. Diagnosis and treatment can be complicated by co-ingestion of other drugs (frequency >80%).
General/Chronic: as for intoxication.
Withdrawal: psychological support and counselling.

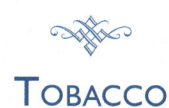

Tobacco

Tobacco is produced from the tobacco plant – *Nicotiana tabacum*. Nicotine is the chief addictive ingredient in tobacco.

Principal Drugs and Derivatives

The content of tobacco smoke is complex. About 500 different compounds have been identified. The main pharmacologically active ingredients are nicotine and tars. Nicotine is an oily alkaloid. Pure nicotine is extremely poisonous – a dose of 50 mg can cause death within minutes.

Manufacture

Tobacco plants are commercially cultivated and harvested worldwide. Synthetic nicotine (SN) e-cigarettes have emerged on the market as an alternative to tobacco-derived nicotine (TDN) vaping products.

Common Street Names

Ciggies, tabs, roll-ups, fags, smokes, gaspers.

Mechanism of Action

Nicotine is both a stimulant and a sedative, with effects on the central nervous and voluntary and involuntary nervous systems that are dose dependent. In the doses used in smoking, nicotine causes release of catecholamines, serotonin, antidiuretic hormone, corticotrophin and growth

DOI: 10.4324/9781003381730-33

hormone. Nicotine inhaled as smoke will reach the brain within 1 min. Its effects on the body last for about 30 min. It is excreted in urine after metabolism to inert substances. Cotinine, another component of tobacco but also a metabolite of nicotine, is sometimes used as a marker for tobacco use.

Medical Uses

None.

Legal Status

Tobacco products may not be sold to those under 18 years of age in the UK. It is illegal for an adult to buy cigarettes, or for a retailer to sell them if for a person under this age. It is also illegal for adults to buy e-cigarettes or e-liquids for someone under the age of 18. It is illegal to smoke tobacco in enclosed public places, such as restaurants, shops or pubs, under the Health Act 2006 for England and Wales, the Smoking (Northern Ireland) Order 2006 for Northern Ireland and the Smoking, Health and Social Care (Scotland) Act 2005 for Scotland.

Presentation and Methods of Administration

Dried leaves of the tobacco plant may be smoked in cigarettes (manu-factured or 'roll-ups'), cigars, pipes and snuff. One cigarette may con-tain up to 20 mg nicotine, but lower nicotine brands may be as low as 0.5 mg and ultra-low as low as 0.1 mg. Actual nicotine content may bear little relationship to the amount of nicotine ingested. A cigarette may contain up to 15 mg tar, low-tar brands containing considerably less. E-cigarettes and vaping devices are widely available. The leaves may be chewed. Ground-up dried tobacco may be taken as snuff. Snus is a tobacco product and non-tobacco nicotine product consumed by placing a pouch of powdered tobacco leaves or powdered non-tobacco plant fibers under the lip. Waterpipe tobacco (WPT) smoking has surged since the introduction of pre-packaged flavored and sweet-ened WPT.

Symptoms and Signs

Acute Intoxication

Physical: tachycardia, hypertension, sore throat, sore eyes and tremor. Seizures and arrhythmias have been documented with e-cigarettes.
Psychological: some individuals feel more alert and some feel more tranquil.

General/Chronic

Physical: physical dependence develops rapidly (within days). Long-term smoking is associated with a large range of diseases and illnesses including lung cancer, atherosclerosis (manifest as angina, myocardial infarction, cerebrovascular accidents or peripheral vascular disease), bronchitis, peptic ulcers, reduced fertility (females), complications of pregnancy (including smaller babies), poor oral health and cancers of the mouth and throat. Children of female smokers may be shorter and have delayed intellectual development. All these risks increase the longer the individual has smoked. The risks vary according to the type of use (e.g. cigarettes versus pipes) and the method of use (e.g. inhaling versus not inhaling). Stopping smoking will eventually decrease the risk.
Psychological: psychological dependence is marked.

Cessation/Withdrawal

A withdrawal syndrome develops with the individual initially experiencing fatigue, shortness of breath and headache, and longer-term agitation, irritability and depression. Many individuals become preoccupied with the absence of smoking. Weight gain may be observed because of a reduction in metabolic rate and 'comfort' eating.

Treatment

Intoxication: no specific treatment.
General/chronic: the ease (or not) of cessation of smoking varies with each individual. Some individuals may stop without support, but most

require help. Tapered nicotine replacement therapy (NRT), using nicotine-supplying gum, lozenges, sublingual tablets, skin patches or e-cigarettes, may be useful. Drugs such as varenicline (a selective nicotine receptor partial agonist) used in conjunction with NRT have been trialed with some effect. Anxiolytic drugs, counselling, hypnotherapy and acupuncture all have their place in the management of those experiencing difficulties.

Withdrawal: no specific treatment, except NRT.

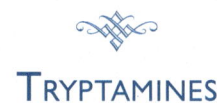

TRYPTAMINES

Principal Drugs and Derivatives

This is a very broad category of drugs including endogenous compounds such as serotonin (5-hydroxytryptamine) and melatonin, naturally occurring compounds such as psilocybin, bufotenine (5-hydroxydimethyltryptamine), mitragynine, DMT (dimethyltryptamine) and 5-MeO-DMT (5-methoxy-dimethyltryptamine), psilocin (4-hydroxy-N, N-dimethyltryptamine and synthetic drugs including AMT (α-methyltryptamine), 5-MeO-DALT (N,N-diallyl-5-methoxytryptamine) and 5-methoxy-*N*, *N*-diisopropyl-tryptamine. They are derived from tryptophan.

Manufacture

Psilocybin occurs naturally in more than 200 species of mushrooms belonging to the genus *Psilocybe*. One of the most common species is *P. semilanceata*, which occurs in Europe and the Americas. *P. cubensis* occurs in the Americas, Asia and Australasia.

Bufotenine occurs as a secretion in cane toads including *Bufo vulgaris* and *B. viridis*. The drug also occurs in the seeds of a number of plants including *Anadenanthera peregrine* and *A. columbrina*, which are both large trees growing in South America. Other parts of the plants contain other tryptamines.

Mitragynine occurs naturally in the plant Mitragyna speciosa.

Many tryptamines may also be manufactured synthetically.

Common Street Names

Psilocybe mushrooms: magic mushrooms, shrooms, caps.

DOI: 10.4324/9781003381730-34

Bufotenine: toad, love stones.
Mitragynine: kratom.
5-Methoxy-N, N-diisopropyltryptamine: foxy, foxy methoxy
5-methoxydimethyltryptamine: O-DMS, alpha-O, alpha and O-DMS.
N,N-diallyl-5-methoxytryptamine: rockstar, green-beans, 5-MED, jungles.

Mechanism of Action

Some naturally occurring tryptamines are neurotransmitters (e.g. serotonin, melatonin and bufotenine), most are psychoactive hallucinogens found in plants, fungi and animals. Interaction with serotonin receptors in the brain produces alteration of auditory and visual perception.

These drugs are absorbed by the gastrointestinal tract, with an effect within 20 min of ingestion. DMT is reported to have no activity if taken orally and requires injection or coadministration with a compound to prevent first-pass metabolism.

Oral dosage of the synthetically produced tryptamines can vary from 5 mg to 100 mg, but varies significantly between similar compounds and the route of ingestion, so care is needed to avoid excessive dosage. 2 mg AMT smoked is an effective dose. Large dosages of some drugs may produce effects lasting more than 24 h. Half-lives have not been established.

Medical Uses

None currently although there are suggestions certain compounds should be explored for medical use.

Legal Status

Tryptamines are classified as class A under the Misuse of Drugs Act 1971 and under schedule 1 of the Misuse of Drugs Regulations 2001.

Presentation and Methods of Administration

Powders, capsules, tablets, paper squares. Taken orally or by snorting.

Psilocybe mushrooms may be ingested as picked fresh or dried. A typical dose of fresh mushrooms would be 10–20 mushrooms but fewer for dried specimens.

Bufo toads may be licked ('toad-licking') but the dose is very variable. Many indigenous people use preparations of tryptamines in rituals, sometimes as snuffs for nasal inhalation or drinks. Again the dosage is variable.

Symptoms and Signs

Acute Intoxication

Physical: very varied effects can include nausea, vomiting, dizziness, and psychedelic effects including visual, temporal and auditory hallucinations. The use of mushrooms in single high doses is linked to medical emergencies. Tachycardia, tachypnoea and hypertension may be present. Trismus, sweating, diarrhoea, sialorrhoea, palpitations and mydriasis have all been reported. Fatality has been reported.
Psychological: psychedelic effects, sometimes in waves. Higher doses can result in disorientation, irrational behaviour, confusion, dysphoria, fear, delusions, paranoia and psychosis.

General/Chronic

Multiple doses of psilocybin in the same session or its combination with other substances are linked to the occurrence of long-term negative outcomes.

Driving

All likely to be incompatible with driving a motor vehicle but no known studies. Cases have been reported.

Treatment

Intoxication: nil – unless complications develop. Then supportive with monitoring of vital signs in hospital setting; intravenous benzodiazepines may be appropriate.

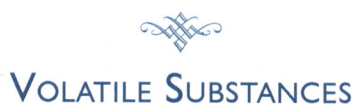

VOLATILE SUBSTANCES

Principal Drugs

Toluene, acetone, butane, fluorocarbons, propane, trichloroethylene, tri-chloroethane ethyl acetate, xylenes.

Manufacture

Laboratory/factory production.

Common Street Names

Gases, solvents, thinners.

Medical Uses

Apart from the anaesthetic agents such as nitrous oxide there are no medical uses for these substances.

Mechanism of Action

The solvents are rapidly absorbed through the lungs and pass into the bloodstream. They are highly lipid soluble, with effects being experienced within minutes. These generally last less than an hour unless repetitive inhalation occurs.

DOI: 10.4324/9781003381730-35

Legal Status

Widely available in shops. It is an offence to sell any intoxicating substances to a person under the age of 18, where the retailer may reasonably believe that the product will be used for intoxication.

Presentation and Methods of Administration

A variety of compounds can be subject to misuse and the process is commonly referred to as volatile substance abuse (VSA). Compounds involved may include: solvents in adhesives (glue) such as toluene, ethyl acetate, hexane, xylenes; acetone in nail polish; fuel gases such as butane, isobutane and propane; petrol; fluorocarbons in aerosols; dry-cleaning and degreasing agents such as trichloroethylene, tetrachloroethylene, dichloromethane and trichloroethane; ozone-benign aerosol propellants such as halon; propellants in some inhalers; anaesthetic agents such as nitrous oxide or halothane.

VSA can be defined as the inhalation of such fumes in order to achieve intoxication. Vapours or gases are inhaled through the nose or mouth with the method depending on the substance misused, e.g. some products can be sniffed directly from their containers, or glue may be put in a plastic bag for inhalation ('huffing'); direct injection of lighter refills, via depression of the nozzle between the teeth, is a particularly dangerous method of ingestion.

Symptoms and Signs

Acute Intoxication

Physical: the solvent smell may be apparent on the breath, hands and clothing; nasal sores, burns, adhesive marks and 'glue-sniffer's rash' (perioral eczema) may be seen. Nausea, vomiting, sneezing, coughing and diarrhoea may occur. High doses may result in depression of the central nervous system with drowsiness, slurred speech, nystagmus, ataxia, visual disturbances and coma.

Dependence and Convulsions

Sudden death is a recognised complication of volatile solvent use and may occur during exposure or the post-exposure period, or result from trauma or asphyxia secondary to intoxication. Death may result from anoxia, respiratory depression, vagal inhibition and cardiac dysrhythmias. Dysrhythmias may be difficult to treat and the risk remains for several hours after inhalation. In pregnancy usage may lead to neonatal depression and there is a possibility of teratogenicity. After the acute effects wear off, there may be drowsiness and headaches with poor concentration, which may last for up to a day or so.

Psychological: euphoria with excitatory effects secondary to disinhibition (similar to alcohol but the effects occur more quickly). With increasing dosage there may be perceptual disturbances, hallucinations and delusions.

Chronic

The drugs may result in fatigue, memory impairment with poor concentration, weight loss and depression. The effects are dependent on substance abused as well as the duration and intensity of abuse. Tolerance can develop if the misuse occurs over a prolonged period but a physical dependence syndrome is not a problem although psychological dependence may occur. Very long-term misuse may result in liver or renal failure, liver tumours, bone marrow depression, anaemia and nervous system involvement, including cerebellar disease, dementia and peripheral neuropathy. Perioral eczema and upper respiratory tract problems may occur with chronic misuse.

Driving

Driving immediately after VSA is unlikely, although attempts may be made before the abuser's cognition and coordination have returned to normal and this would be potentially unlawful and dangerous. Most road traffic offences involve people who are 'in charge' of a motor vehicle rather than actually driving.

Treatment

There are no specific treatments other than removal of the source material where possible and removal of the person from any contaminated atmosphere. Many effects are reversible on cessation of solvent misuse, except when the product is highly toxic as with leaded petrol where brain damage has occurred through lead poisoning.

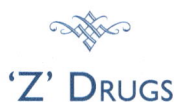

'Z' Drugs

Principal Drugs

Zaleplon, zolpidem, zopiclone, eszopiclone

Common Street Names

Zombie, sleep-easy, zim, zimmies, zimmers.

Mechanism of Action

Sedative–hypnotic drugs that depress the central nervous system.

Medical Uses

These are non-benzodiazepine hypnotic drugs that act on the benzodiazepine receptors. Zaleplon is very short acting, and zopiclone and zolpidem are short acting. The half-life of zaleplon is 1 h, zolpidem 1.5–4.5 h, zopiclone 3.5–6.5 h, eszopiclone ~ 6.0h. Zaleplon is recommended for a maximum of 2 weeks' use, and zolpidem and zopiclone for up to 4 weeks.

Legal Status

These drugs are prescription-only medicines and are now all controlled under the Misuse of Drugs Act 1971 as class C drugs.

Presentation and Methods of Administration

Tablets and capsules.

DOI: 10.4324/9781003381730-36

Symptoms and Signs

Acute Intoxication

Physical: sedation, with increasing doses; slurred speech, visual disturbances, loss of coordination, dysphoria, respiratory depression. All of these drugs are relatively safe in overdosage unless taken in combination with other drugs or alcohol. Sulfhaemoglobinaemia has been reported with high dose zopiclone. A bitter or metallic taste may accompany the use of eszopiclone.

Psychological: anxiolytic, impairment of memory and cognition, hallucinations, parasomnia, somnambulism.

Chronic

Sedative–hypnotic drugs may cause physical and psychological dependence and an abstinence syndrome, although such effects are reported to be rare with the 'Z' drugs unless larger than prescribed dosage is taken.

Withdrawal effects, when they occur, start within 24 h with anxiety, rebound insomnia, tremors, tachycardia and seizures having been reported. There is an increased risk of fatality when co-prescribed with other drugs such as gabapentin.

Driving

All 'Z' drugs have the potential to impair driving ability due to their sedative effects. If taken as prescribed there are likely to be few residual effects the next morning, although patients should be warned of the possibility. Driving within a few hours of taking the drugs is likely to cause decrement of driving ability with poor concentration and coordination although the effects on cognition remain unclear. Particular care is required when prescribing to the elderly.

Treatment

Supportive measures are gastric lavage if recent overdose; flumazenil may be used to reverse sedation in the hospital environment.

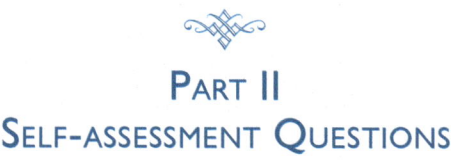

Part II
Self-assessment Questions

Alcohol

1. What drug would you use to treat alcohol withdrawal in police custody and why?
2. How many units are there in:

   a. One pint of beer (568 mL) 4% ABV

   b. A 175 mL glass of red wine, 13.5% ABV

Aminoindanes, Indoles and Benzofurans

1. What is MDAI?
2. How is it used?

Amphetamine-type Stimulants

1. Why is methamphetamine more dangerous than amphetamine?
2. What is 'stacking' and why can this lead to death?

Barbiturates

1. List some better alternatives to barbiturates for treating insomnia
2. Why are barbiturates, other than phenobarbitone, so dangerous?

DOI: 10.4324/9781003381730-37

Benzodiazepines

1. How can different benzodiazepines be classified?
2. What is 'benzo dope'?
3. What are the symptoms and signs of withdrawal from benzodiazepines?

Cannabis

1. Why is 'skunk' more dangerous than traditional herbal cannabis?
2. What is 'honey-oil'?
3. What signs may you see if a driver has a 'condition' due to the drug cannabis?

Cocaine

1. What is meant by 'binging' on cocaine?
2. What is the relationship between cocaine hydrochloride and 'crack' cocaine?
3. What signs may you see if an individual is suffering with ABD resulting from the use of cocaine?

Ecstasy

1. How is 'ecstasy' normally taken?
2. What are the symptoms and signs of excessive MDMA ingestion?

Gabapentinoids

1. Name two gabapentinoids.
2. Which of the two is most likely to be misused and why?
3. How would you treat withdrawal from gabapentinoids?

γ-Hydroxybutyrate and Related Compounds

1. What makes prior use of GHB difficult to detect in a living subject?
2. Why is GHB a dangerous drug?
3. What are the symptoms and signs of withdrawal and how would you treat withdrawal?

Ketamine

1. List the various methods by which ketamine can be misused.
2. Describe the suite of effects which gives ketamine a unique pharmacodynamic profile.

Khat

1. How is khat used traditionally?
2. What effects are produced?

LSD

1. From where does lysergic acid derive?
2. How is LSD metabolised?
3. Provide examples of psychological effects of LSD.

Nitrites

1. What type of poisoning can alkyl nitrite treat?
2. Are nitrites controlled under the Misuse of Drugs Act 1971?
3. How may nitrites be used to reduce the risks of penetrative sex?

Nitrous Oxide

1. What medical uses are there for nitrous oxide?
2. What are the adverse medical effects of nitrous oxide use?
3. What management is required for the adverse medical effects of nitrous oxide?

Opiates/Opioids

1. How can an overdose of an opiate or opioid drug be treated?
2. Detail two methods by which heroin can be abused.
3. Why are fentanyls and nitazenes so dangerous?

Phencyclidine

1. What type of drug is phencyclidine?
2. What are the signs and symptoms of phencyclidine use?
3. Is phencyclidine a drug of dependence?

Phenylethylamines

1. Give three examples of phenylethylamines.
2. In what form may phenylethylamine be presented?
3. What are the physical signs of phenylethylamine use?

Piperazines

1. When may piperazines be used in medical settings?
2. How are piperazines classified under the Misuse of Drugs Act 1971?
3. Name three adverse effect of piperazine use.

Pipradrols

1. What is the mechanism of action of pipradrols?
2. Name four physical signs of pipradrol use.
3. What class and schedule are pipradrols controlled under?

Synthetic Cannabinoids

1. What is the mechanism of action of synthetic cannabinoids?
2. Do synthetic cannabinoids have medical uses?
3. What neurological complications can be caused by synthetic cannabinoids?

Synthetic Cathinones

1. From what plant are cathinones derived?
2. Do synthetic cathinones have medical uses?
3. Name four signs of high dose synthetic cathinone intoxication.

Tobacco

1. What is the most clinically significant ingredient in tobacco?
2. Can tobacco products be sold to 17-year-olds?
3. What techniques or methods can be used to assist in cessation of smoking?

Tryptamines

1. Provide two examples each of natural tryptamines and synthetic tryptamines.
2. Name four signs of tryptamine intoxication.
3. How are tryptamines classed and scheduled under (respectively) the Misuse of Drugs Act 1971 and the Misuse of Drugs Regulations 2001?

Volatile Substances

1. Provide three examples of domestic products that may be subject to volatile substance abuse.
2. Provide four modes of death which can be caused by volatile substance abuse.
3. Provide three examples of signs particularly associated with volatile substance abuse.

'Z' Drugs

1. What are the main medical indications for the use of 'Z' drugs?
2. Can 'Z' drugs be bought over the counter?
3. Provide three symptoms of withdrawal from 'Z' drugs.

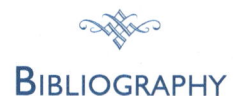

BIBLIOGRAPHY

Part I

Advisory Council for the Misuse of Drugs, 2019. *Ageing Cohort of Drug Users.* https://assets.publishing.service.gov.uk/media/5d037c2ee-5274a0b8016b395/Ageing_cohort_of_drug_users.pdf

Cole C, Jones L, McVeigh J, Kicman A, Syed Q, Bellis M. Adulterants in illicit drugs: a review of empirical evidence. *Drug Test Anal* 2011 Feb;**3**(2): 89–96. doi: 10.1002/dta.220. Epub 2010 Dec 29. PMID: 21322119.

Department of Health & Social Care, January 2013. *The Medical Care of Suspected Internal Drug Traffickers – Independent Report of the Chief Medical Officer's Expert Group.* https://assets.publishing.service.gov.uk/government/uploads/system/uploads/attachment_data/file/213336/SIDT-Report-FINAL.pdf

Eide D, Lobmaier P, Clausen T. Who is using take-home naloxone? An examination of supersavers. *Harm Reduct J* 2022 Jun 18;**19**(1):65. doi: 10.1186/s12954-022-00647-z.

EMCDDA, October 2023. Spotlight on drug checking. https://www.euda.europa.eu/spotlights/spotlight-drug-checking_en

Faculty of Forensic and Legal Medicine, 2024. *Guidelines for Doctors Asked to Perform Intimate Body Searches.* London: FFLM.

Faculty of Forensic and Legal Medicine, 2024. *Intimate Searches in Police Custody Flowchart.* London: FFLM.

Faculty of Forensic and Legal Medicine, 2024. *Acute Behavioural Disturbance: Guidelines on Management in Police Custody.* London: FFLM.

Home Office, 2024. *Understanding and Tackling Spiking.* https://assets.publishing.service.gov.uk/media/663b30dd4d8bb7378fb6c340/E02885674_Statutory_Report_on_Spiking_Accessible.pdf

House of Commons Home Affairs Committee, August 2023. *Drugs.* Third Report of Session 2022–23. 31 August 2023. https://publications.parliament.uk/pa/cm5803/cmselect/cmhaff/198/report.html

Norfolk GA The fatal case of a cocaine body-stuffer and a literature review – towards evidence-based management. *Journal of Forensic and Legal Medicine* 2007;**14**(1):49–52.

Office for National Statistics (ONS), 19 December 2023, ONS website, statistical bulletin. https://www.ons.gov.uk/peoplepopulationandcommunity/birthsdeathsandmarriages/deaths/bulletins/deathsrelatedtodrugpoisoninginenglandandwales/2022registrations

Ouellette RR, Selino S, Kong G. Electronic nicotine delivery systems and e-liquid modifications to vape cannabis depicted in online videos. *JAMA Netw Open* 2023 Nov;6(11): e2341075. Published online 2023 Nov 2.

Nitro L, Pipolo C, Fadda GL et al. Distribution of cocaine-induced midline destructive lesions: systematic review and classification. *Eur Arch Otorhinolaryngol* 2022;279(7):3257–3267. Published online 2022 Feb 9. doi: 10.1007/s00405-022-07290-1PMCID: PMC9130192.

Royal College of Emergency Medicine, December 2020. *Best Practice Guideline. Management of Suspected Internal Drug Trafficker (SIDT)*. https://rcem.ac.uk/wp-content/uploads/2021/10/Management_of_Suspected_Internal_Drug_Trafficker_December_2020.pdf

Royal College of Emergency Medicine, October 2023. *Best Practice Guideline. Acute Behavioural Disturbance in Emergency Departments*. https://rcem.ac.uk/wp-content/uploads/2023/10/Acute_Behavioural_Disturbance_in_Emergency_Departments_Oct2023_V2.pdf

Royal College of Psychiatrists, 2018. *Our Invisible Addicts College Report CR 211*. www.rcpsych.ac.uk

Royal College of Psychiatrists and Faculty of Forensic and Legal Medicine, 2020. *Detainees with Substance Use Disorders in Police Custody. Guidelines for Clinical Management*, fifth edition. College report CR 227. https://fflm.ac.uk/resources/publications/detainees-with-substance-use-disorders-in-police-custody-guidelines-for-clinical-management-5th-edition/

UK Health Security Agency, Public Health Agency Northern Ireland, Public Health Scotland and Public Health Wales, March 2023. *Shooting Up: Infections and Other Injecting-related Harms Among People Who Inject Drugs in the UK*. Data to end of 2021. London: UK Health Security Agency.

Part II

Alcohol

Borkenstein RF, Crowther FR, Shumate RP, et al. The role of the drinking driver in traffic accidents (The Grand Rapids Study). *Blutalkohol* 1974;11(suppl 1):1–132.

Department of Health, 2016. *UK Chief Medical Officers' Alcohol Guidelines Review: Summary of the proposed new guidelines*. https://assets.publishing.service.gov.uk/government/uploads/system/uploads/attachment_data/file/489795/summary.pdf

Jones AW. Alcohol, its absorption, distribution, metabolism, and excretion in the body and pharmacokinetic calculations. *WIREs Forensic Sci* 2019;e1340. https://doi.org/10.1002/wfs2.1340

Jones AW, Andersson L. Influence of age, gender and blood-alcohol concentration on the rate of disappearance rate of alcohol from blood in drinking drivers. *J Forensic Sci* 1996;41(6):922–926.

Krüger HP, Kazenwadel J, Volirath M, et al. Grand Rapids effects revisited: accidents, alcohol and risk. In: *Alcohol, Drugs, and Traffic Safety:* proceedings of the 13th International Conference on Alcohol, Drugs and Traffic Safety, Adelaide. Adelaide, Australia: NHMRC Road Accident Research Unit, 1995: 222–230.

Martin CS, Moss HB. Measurement of acute tolerance to alcohol in human subjects. *Alc Clin Exp Res* 1993;17:211–216.

Royal College of Psychiatrists & Faculty of Forensic and Legal Medicine, 2020. *Detainees with Substance Use Disorders in Police Custody: Guidelines for Clinical Management,* fifth edition. College report CR 227. https://fflm. ac.uk/resources/publications/detainees-with-substance-use-disorders-in-police-custody-guidelines-for-clinical-management-5th-edition/

Aminoindanes, Indoles and Benzofurans

Corkery JM, Elliott S, Schifano F et al. MDAI (5,6-methylenedioxy-2-aminoindane; 6,7-dihydro-5H-cyclopental[f][1,3]benzodioxol-6-amine; 'sparkle'; 'mindy') toxicity; a brief overview and update. *Hum Psychopharmacol Clin Exp* 2013;28:345–355.

Gallagher CT, Assi S, Stair JL, et al. 5,6-Methylenedioxy-2-aminoindane: from laboratory curiosity to 'legal high'. *Hum Psychopharmacol* 2012;27: 106–12.

Iversen L, Gibbons S, Treble R et al. Neurochemical profiles of some novel psychoactive substances. *Eur J Pharmacol* 2013;700:147–51.

Iversen L, White M, Treble R. Designer psychostimulants: pharmacology and differences. *Neuropharmacology* 2014 Jan 15. http://dx.doi.org/10.1016/j. neuropharm.

Jebadurai J, Schifano F, Deluca P. Recreational use of 1-(2-naphthyl)-2-(1-pyrrolidinyl)-1-pentanonehydrochloride (NRG-1), 6-(2-aminopropyl) benzofuran (Benzofury/6-APB) and NRG-2 with review of available evidence-based literature. *Hum Psychopharmacol Clin Exp* 2013;28: 356–364.

Oeri HE. Beyond ecstasy: alternative entactogens to 3,4-methylenedioxymethamphetamine with potential applications in psychotherapy. *J Psychopharmacol* 2021 May;35(5):512–536. doi: 10.1177/0269881120920420. Epub 2020 Sep 10.

Pinterova N, Horsley RR, Palenicek T. Synthetic Aminoindanes: a summary of existing knowledge. *Front. Psychiatry* 2017;**8**:236.

Seetohul LN, Maskell PD, De Paoli G, et al. Deaths associated with new designer drug 5-IT. *BMJ* 2012;**345**:e5625.

Shulgin AT, Shulgin A., 1997. *TiHKAL −The Continuation.* Berkeley, CA: Transform Press.

Simmler LD, Rickli A, Schramm Y et al. Pharmacological profiles of aminoindanes, piperazines and pipradrol derivatives. *Biochem Pharmacol* 2014;**88**:237–244.

UNODC Laboratory and Scientific Service. Portals. Aminoindanes. https://www.unodc.org/LSS/SubstanceGroup/Details/8fd64573-c567-4734-a258-76d1d95dca25.

Vari MR, Pichini S, Giorgetti R et al. New psychoactive substances − synthetic stimulants. *WIREs Forensic Sci* 2019;**1**:e1197.

Amphetamine-type Stimulants

Al-Imam A, Santacroce R, Roman-Urrestarazu A et al. Captagon: use and trade in the Middle East. *Hum Psychopharmacol Clin Exp* 2017; **32**:e2548

Barkholtz HM, Hadzima R, Miles A. Pharmacology of R-(-)-methamphetamine in humans: a systematic review of the literature. *ACS Pharmacol Transl Sci* 2023;**6**:914–924.

Caldicott DGE, Edwards NA, Kruys A, et al. Dancing with 'death': *p*-methoxyamphetamine overdose and its acute management. *Clin Toxicol* 2003;**41**:143–154.

De laTorre R, Farré M, Navarro M, Pacifici R, Zuccaro P, Pichini S. Clinical pharmacokinetics of amfetamine and related substances. *Clin Pharmacokinet* 2004;**43**:157–185.

Ellinwood EH, Nikaido AM. Stimulant induced impairment: a perspective across dose and duration of use. *Alcohol Drugs Driv* 1987;**3**:19–24.

Emonson L, Vanderbeek RD. The use of amphetamines in US Air Force tactical operations during Desert Shield and Storm. *Aviat Space Environ Med* 1995;**66**:260–263.

Ermer JC, Pennick M, Frick G. Lisdexamfetamine dimesylate: prodrugdelivery, amphetamine exposure and duration of efficacy. *Clin Drug Investig* 2016;**36**:341–356.

European Monitoring Centre for Drugs and Drug Addiction and Europol, 2019. *Methamphetamine in Europe, EMCDDA-Europol Threat Assessment.* Luxembourg: Publications Office of the European Union.

Gjerde H, Christophersen AS, Morland J. Amphetamine and drugged driving. *J Traffic Med* 1992;**20**:21–26.

Harris D, Batki SL. Stimulant psychosis: symptom profile and acute clinical course. *Am J Addict* 2000;**9**:28–37.

Hart JB, Wallace J. The adverse effects of amphetamines. *Clin Toxicol* 1975;**8**:179–190.

Hurst PM. Amphetamines and driving. *Alcohol Drugs Driv* 1987;**3**:13–16.

Johansen SS, Hansen AC, Müller IB, et al. Three fatal cases of PMA and PMMA poisoning in Denmark. *J Analyt Toxicol* 2003;**27**:253–256.

Kolaczynska K, Luethi D, Trachsel D et al. Receptor interaction profiles of 4-alkoxy-substituted 2,5-dimethoxyphenethylamines and related amphetamines. *Front Pharmacol* 2019;**10**:1423.

Logan BK. Methamphetamine and driving impairment. *J Forensic Sci* 1996;**41**:457–464.

Logan BK. Methamphetamine – effects on human performance and behavior. *Forensic Sci Rev* 2002;**14**:133–151.

Mackay A, Downey LA, Arunogiri S, Ogeil RP, Hayley AC. Trait anger as a predictor of dangerous driving behaviour amongst people who use methamphetamine. *Accid Anal Prev* 2024 Sep;**204**:107634. doi: 10.1016/j.aap.2024.107634. Epub 2024 May 24.

Silber BY, Papafotiou K, Croft RJ, et al. An evaluation of the sensitivity of the standardised field sobriety tests to detect the presence of amphetamine. *Psychopharmacology* 2005;**182**:153–159.

Simon MW, Olsen HA, Hoyte O et al. Clinical effects of psychedelic substances reported to United States poison centers: 2012 to 2022. *Ann Emerg Med* 2024 1August:S0196–0644(24)00384-6. doi: 10.1016/j.annemergmed.2024.06.025.

Smith ME, Farah MJ. Are prescription stimulants 'smart pills'? The epidemiology and cognitive neuroscience of prescription stimulant use by normal healthy individuals. *Psychol Bull* 2011;**137**:717–741.

Steinkellner T, Freissmuth M, Sitte H et al. The ugly side of amphetamines: short- and long-term toxicity of 3,4-methylenedioxymethamphetamine (MDMA, 'ecstasy'), methamphetamine and d-amphetamine. *Biol Chem* 2011;**392**:103–115.

Vevelstad M, Øestad EL, Middelkoop G, et al. The PMMA epidemic in Norway: comparison of fatal and non-fatal intoxications. *Forensic Sci Int* 2012;**219**:151–157.

Barbiturates

Betts TA, Clayton AB, Mackay GM. Effects of four commonly used tranquillizers on low-speed driving performance tests. *BMJ* 1972;**4**:580–584.

Brodie MJ, Kwan P. Current position of phenobarbital in epilepsy and its future. *Epilepsia* 2012;**53**(suppl 8):40–46.

Coupey SM. Barbiturates. *Pediatr Rev* 1987;**18**:260–264.

Frohnapple C, Nobay F, Acquisto NM, 2024. Barbiturates. *Encyclopedia of Toxicology* (fourth edition) Volume 1. Elsevier, pages 903–910.

Johns MW. Sleep and hypnotic drugs. *Drugs* 1975;**9**:448–478.

Wang M, Falank C, Simboli V, Ontengco JB, Spurling B, Rappold J, Chung B, Smith KE. 'Should we phenobarb-it-all?' A phenobarbital-based protocol for non-intensive care unit trauma patients at high risk of or experiencing alcohol withdrawal. *Am Surg* 2024 Jun;**90**(6):1531–1539. doi: 10.1177/00031348241244639.

Yeakel JK, Logan BK. Butalbital and driving impairment. *J Forensic Sci* 2013;**58**:941–945.

Benzodiazepines

Barbone F, McMahon AD, Davey PG, et al. Association of road-traffic accidents with benzodiazepine use. *Lancet* 1998;**352**:1331–1336.

Berghaus G, Sticht G, Grellner W, Lenz D, Naumann Th, Wiesenmüller S., 2010. Meta-analysis of empirical studies concerning the effects of medicines and illegal drugs including pharmacokinetics on safe driving. *Driving under the Influence of Drugs, Alcohol and Medicines (DRUID)*. Brussels: European Commission, Directorate-General for Energy and Transport.

Brunetti P, Giorgetti R, Tagliabracci A et al. Designer benzodiazepines: a review of toxicology and public health risks. *Pharmaceuticals* 2021;**14**;560.

Busardo FP, Di Trana A, Montanari E et al. Is etizolam a safe medication? Effects on psychomotor performance at therapeutic dosages of a newly abused psychoactive substance. *Forensic Sci Int.* 2019;**301**;137–141.

Dassanayake T, Michie P, Carter G, Jones A. Effects of benzodiazepines, antidepressants and opioids on driving: a systematic review and meta-analysis of epidemiological and experimental evidence. *Drug Saf* 2011 Feb 1;**34**(2):125–156. doi: 10.2165/11539050-000000000-00000.

Drummer OH. Benzodiazepines – effects on human performance and behaviour. *Forensic Sci Rev* 2008;**14**:2–14.

European Monitoring Centre for Drugs and Drug Addiction (2021), *New benzodiazepines in Europe –a review.* Luxembourg: Publications Office of the European Union.

Greenblatt DJ. Pharmacology of benzodiazepine hypnotics. *J Clin Psychiatry* 1992;**53**:7–13.

Hojer J, Baehrendtz S, Gustaffson L. Benzodiazepine poisoning: experience of 702 admissions to an intensive care unit during a 14-year period. *J Intern Med* 1989;**226**:117–122.

Kelly E, Darke S, Ross JA. Review of drug use and driving: epidemiology, impairment, risk factors, and risk perceptions. *Drug Alcohol Rev* 2004;**23**:319–344.

Kurtz SP, Surratt HL, Levi-Minzi MA, et al. Benzodiazepine dependence among multidrug users in the club scene. *Drug Alcohol Depend* 2011;**119**:99–105.

Lukasik-Glebocka M, Sommerfeld K, Tezyk A et al. Flubromazolam – a new life-threatening designer benzodiazepine. *Clin Toxicol* 2016;**54**;66–68.

Maskell PD, De Paoli G, Nitin Seetohul L, et al. Phenazepam: the drug that came in from the cold. *J Forensic Legal Med* 2012;**19**:122–125.

Ntoupa P-SA, Papoutsis II, Dona AA et al. A fluorine turns a medicinal benzodiazepine into NPS: the case of flualprazolam. *Forensic Toxicol* 2021;**39**:368–376.

Rapoport MJ, Lanctôt KL, Streiner DL, et al. Benzodiazepine use and driving: a meta-analysis. *J Clin Psychiatry* 2009;**70**:663–673.

Smink BE, Egberts AC, Lusthof KJ, et al. The relationship between benzodiazepine use and traffic accidents: a systematic literature review. *CNS Drugs* 2010;**24**:639–653.

Smink BE, Lusthof KJ, de Grier JJ, et al. The relation between the blood benzodiazepine concentration and performance in suspected impaired drivers. *J Forensic Legal Med* 2008;**15**:483–488.

Cannabis

Asbridge M, Hayden JA, Cartwright JL. Acute cannabis consumption and motor vehicle collision risk: systematic review of observational studies and meta-analysis. *BMJ* 2012;**344**:e536.

Bell C, Slim J, Flaten HK et al. Butane hash oil burns associated with marijuana liberalization in Colorado. *J Med Toxicol* 2015;**11**;422–425.

Berghaus G, Sticht G, Grellner W, Lenz D, Naumann Th, Wiesenmüller S., 2010. Meta-analysis of empirical studies concerning the effects of medicines and illegal drugs including pharmacokinetics on safe driving. *Driving under the Influence of Drugs, Alcohol and Medicines (DRUID)*. Brussels: European Commission, Directorate-General for Energy and Transport.

Böcker KBE, Gerritsen J, Hunault CC, Kruidenier M, Mensinga TT, Kenemans JL. Cannabis with high D^9-THC contents affects perception and visual selective attention. *Pharmacol Biochem Behav* 2010;**96**:67–74.

Bosker WM, Kuypers KP, Theunissen EL, et al. Medicinal D(9)-tetrahydrocannabinol (dronabinol) impairs on-the-road driving performance of occasional and heavy cannabis users but is not detected in Standard Field Sobriety Tests. *Addiction* 2012;**107**:1837–1844.

Bozman ME, Manoharan SVR, Vasavada T. Marijuana variant of concern: Delta-8-tetrahydrocannabinol (Delta-8-THC, Δ^8-THC). *Psychiatry Res Case Rep* 2022;**1**:100028.

Consroe P, Musty R, Rein J, et al. The perceived effects of smoked cannabis on patients with multiple sclerosis. *Eur Neurol* 1997;**38**:44–48.

Grotenhermen F, Leson G, Berghaus G et al. Developing limits for driving under cannabis. *Addiction* 2007;**12**;1910–1917.

House of Lords, 1998. *Cannabis: Science and Technology.* Ninth Report (accessed 8 August 2023).

Huestis MA. Cannabis (marijuana) – effects on human behavior and performance. *Forensic Sci Rev* 2002;**14**:15–60.

Legare CA, Raup-Konsavage WM, Vrana KE. Therapeutic potential of cannabis, cannabidiol, and cannabinoid-based pharmaceuticals. *Pharmacology* 2022;107(3–4):131–149. doi: 10.1159/000521683.

McCartney D, Arkell TR, Irwin C ct al. Determining the magnitude and duration of acute Δ9-tetrahydrocannabinol (Δ9-THC)-induced driving and cognitive impairment: a systematic and meta-analytic review. *Neurosci & Biobehav Rev* 2021;**126**;175–193.

Moskowitz H. Marijuana and driving. *Acc Anal Prevent* 1985;**17**:323–345.

Murray JB. Marijuana's effects on human cognitive functions, psychomotor functions, and personality. *J Gen Psychol* 1985;**113**:23–55.

Papafotiou K, Carter JD, Stough C. The relationship between performance on the standardised field sobriety tests, driving performance and the level of delta-9-tetrahydrocannabinol (THC) in blood. *Forensic Sci Int* 2005;**155**:172–178.

Potter DJ, Clark P, Brown MB. Potency of delta (9)-THC and other cannabinoids in cannabis in England in 2005: implications for psychoactivity and pharmacology. *J Forensic Sci* 2008;**53**:90–94.

Sexton BF, Tunbridge RJ, Brook-Carter N, Jackson PG, Wright K, Stark MM, Englehart K., 2000. *The Influence of Cannabis on Driving.* TRL Report 477, TRL Ltd for the Road Safety Division, DETR.

Sexton BF, Tunbridge RJ, Board A, Jackson PG, Wright K, Stark MM, Englehart K., 2002. *The Influence of Cannabis and Alcohol on Driving.* TRL Report 543, TRL Ltd for the Road Safety Division Department of Transport.

Spindle TR, Martin EL, Grabenauer M et al. Assessment of cognitive and psychomotor impairment, subjective effects, and blood THC concentrations following acute administration of oral and vaporized cannabis. *J Psychopharmacol* 2021;**35**:786–803.

Thomas H. Psychiatric symptoms in cannabis users. *Br J Psychiatry* 1993;**163**:141–149.

Ward NJ, Dye L.,1999. *Cannabis and Driving – A Review of the Literature and Commentary.* UK DETR Road Safety Research Report No.12. London: DETR.

Cocaine

Awtry EH, Philippides GJ. Alcoholic and cocaine-associated cardiomyopathies. *Prog Cardiovasc Dis* 2010;**52**:289–299.

Benowitz NL. Clinical pharmacology and toxicology of cocaine. *Pharmacol Toxicol* 1993;**72**:3–12.

Brookoff D, Cook CS, Williams C, et al. Testing reckless drivers for cocaine and marijuana. *N Engl J Med* 1994;**331**:518–22.

Cone EJ. Pharmacokinetics and pharmacodynamics of cocaine. *J Analyt Toxicol* 1995;**19**:459–478.

Czermainski FR, Lopes FM, Ornell F et al. Concurrent use of alcohol and crack cocaine is associated with high levels of anger and liability to aggression. *Subst Use & Misuse* 2020;**55**;1660–1666.

Ellinwood EH, Nikaido AM. Stimulant induced impairment: a perspective across dose and duration of use. *Alcohol Drugs Driv* 1987;**3**:19–24.

Gawin FH, Kleber HD. Abstinence symptomatology and psychiatric diagnosis in cocaine abusers. *Arch Gen Psychiatry* 1986;**43**:107–113.

Glossop M, Griffiths P, Powis B, et al. Cocaine: patterns of use, route of administration and severity of dependence. *Br J Psychiatry* 1994;**164**: 660–664.

Isenschmid DS. Cocaine – effects on human performance and behavior. *Forensic Sci Rev* 2002;**14**:62–100.

McCance EF, Price LH, Kosten TR, Jatlow PI. Cocaethylene: pharmacology, physiology and behavioral effects in humans. *J Pharmacol Exp Ther* 1995;**274**:215–233.

Morton WA. Cocaine and psychiatric symptoms. *Prim Care Companion J Clin Psychiatry* 1999;**1**:109–113.

Pennings EJM, Leccese AP, Wolff FA. Effects of concurrent use of alcohol and cocaine. *Addiction* 2002;**97**:773–783.

Pergolizzi J, Breve F, Magnusson P et al. Cocaethylene: when cocaine and alcohol are taken together. *Cureus.* 2022;**14**;e22498.

Ruttenber AJ, Lawler-Hernandez J, Yin M, et al. Fatal excited delirium following cocaine use: epidemiologic findings provide new evidence for mechanisms of cocaine toxicity. *J Forensic Sci* 1997;**42**:25–31.

Siegel RK. Cocaine use and driving behavior. *Alcohol Drugs Driv* 1987;**3**:1–7.

Ecstasy

Bosker WM, Kuypers KPC, Conen S, et al. MDMA (ecstasy) effects on actual driving performance before and after sleep deprivation as function of dose and concentration in blood and oral fluid. *Psychopharmacology* 2012;**222**:367–376.

De Waard D, et al., 2000 A driving simulator study on the effects of MDMA (ecstasy) on driving performance and traffic safety. In: Brookhuis KA, Pernot LMC (eds), *Proceedings of the International Council on Alcohol, Drugs and Traffic Safety*. Stockholm: International Council on Alcohol, Drugs and Traffic Safety.

Jansen KLR. Ecstasy (MDMA) dependence. *Drug Alcohol Depend* 1999; **53**:121–124.

Logan BK, Couper FJ. 3,4-Methylenedioxymethamphetamine – effects on human performance and behavior. *Forensic Sci Rev* 2003; **15**:12–28.

Morgan MJ, McFie L, Fleetwood LH, Robinson JA. Ecstasy (MDMA): are the psychological problems associated with its use reversed by prolonged abstinence? *Psychopharmacology* 2002;**159**:294–303.

Morland J. Toxicity of drug abuse – amphetamine designer drugs (ecstasy): mental effects and consequences of single dose use. *Toxicol Lett* 2000;**112–113**:147–52.

Mounteney J, Griffiths P, Bo A et al. Nine reasons why ecstasy is not quite what it used to be. *Int J Drug Policy* 2018;**51**;36–41.

Rogers G, Elston J, Garside R, Roome C, Taylor R, Younger P, Zawada A, Somerville M. The harmful health effects of recreational ecstasy: a systematic review of observational evidence. *Health Technol Assess* 2009 Jan;13(6): iii–iv, ix–xii, 1–315. doi: 10.3310/hta13050.

Schifano F. Dangerous driving and MDMA ('ecstasy') abuse. *J Serotonin Res* 1995;**1**:53–7.

Schifano F, Oyefeso A, Corkery J, et al. Death rates from ecstasy (MDMA, MDA) and polydrug use in England and Wales 1996–2002. *Hum Psychopharmacol Clin Exp* 2003;**18**:519–524.

Shulgin AT. The background and chemistry of MDMA. *J Psychoact Drugs* 1986;**8**:291–304.

Steele TD, McCann UD, Ricaurte GA. 3,4-methylenedioxymethamphetamine (MDMA, 'ecstasy'): pharmacology and toxicology in animals and humans. *Addiction* 1994;**89**:539–51

Di Trapani L, Eiden C, Mathieu O et al. Life-threatening intoxications related to persistent MDMA (3,4-methylenedioxymethamphetamine) concentrations. *Toxicologie Analytique & Clinique* 2018;**30**:80–83.

Van Amsterdam J, Pennings E, van den Brink W. Fatal and non-fatal health incidents related to recreational ecstasy use. *J Psychopharmacol.* 2020; **34**:591–599.

Vercoulen E, Hondenbrink L. Combining ecstasy and ethanol: higher risk for toxicity? A review. *Crit Rev in Toxicol* 2021;**51**;1–14.

Gabapentinoids

ACMD, 2016. Pregabalin and gabapentin advice. https://assets.publishing.service.gov.uk/media/5a80e1fded915d74e6230fd2/ACMD_Advice_-_Pregabalin_and_gabapentin.pdf

Chiappini S, Schifano F. A decade of gabapentinoid misuse: an analysis of the European Medicines Agency's 'Suspected Adverse Drug Reactions' database CNS drugs 2016;**30**:647–654.

Hagg S, Jonsson AK, Ahiner J. Current evidence on abuse and misuse of gabapentinoids. *Drug Safety* 2020;**43**;1235–1254.

Isoardi KZ, Polkinghorne G, Karris K et al. Pregabalin poisoning and rising recreational use: a retrospective observational series. *Br J Clin Pharmacol* 2020;**86**:2435–2440.

Kalk NJ, Chiu CT, Sadoughi R, Baho H, Williams BD, Taylor D, Copeland CS. Fatalities associated with gabapentinoids in England (2004–2020). *Br J Clin Pharmacol* 2022 Aug;**88**(8):3911–3917. doi: 10.1111/bcp.15352. Epub 2022 Apr 25.

Kriikku P, Wilhelm L, Rintatatlo J et al. Pregabalin serum levels in apprehended drivers. *Forensic Sci Int* 2014;**243**:112–116.

Schifano F. Misuse and abuse of pregabalin and gabapentin: cause for concern? *CNS Drugs* 2014;**28**:491–496.

Tujii T, Kyaw WT, Iwaki H et al. Evaluation of the effect of pregabalin on simulated driving ability using a driving simulator in healthy male volunteers. *Int J Gen Med* 2014;**7**:103–108.

γ-Hydroxybutyrate and Related Compounds

Advisory Council on the Misuse of Drugs, 2020. *An Assessment of the Harms of Gamma-hydroxybutyric Acid (GHB), Gamma-butyrolactone (GBL), and Closely Related Compounds.* London: ACMD. Available from https:// assets.publishing.service.gov.uk/government/uploads/system/uploads/ attachment_data/file/936953/Final_GHBRS_report_20_November_ 2020.pdf (accessed 8 August 2023).

Couper FJ, Marinetti LJ. Gamma-hydroxybutyrate (GHB) – effects on human performance and behavior. *Forensic Sci Rev* 2002;**14**:102–121.

Felmlee MA, Morse BL, Morris ME. γ-Hydroxybutyric acid: pharmacokinetics, pharmacodynamics, and toxicology. *AAPS J* 2022;**23**:22.

Fischer V, Kamphausen T, Buttner A et al. Fatal intoxication with 1,4-butanediol: case report and comprehensive review of the literature. *J. Forensic Sci.* 2023;**68**:1410–1418.

Galloway GP, Frederick-Osborne SL, Seymour R, et al. Abuse and therapeutic potential of gammahydroxybutyric acid. *Alcohol* 2000;**20**:263–269.

Gupta R, Moon G, Bonomo Y, Pastor A. A case of severe and prolonged gamma-hydroxybutyrate (GHB) withdrawal syndrome successfully managed with a slow benzodiazepine and baclofen taper. *Drug Alcohol Rev* 2024 Jul 17. doi: 10.1111/dar.13911.

Jones AW, Holmgren A, Kugelberg FC. Driving under the influence of gamma-hydroxybutyrate (GHB). *Forensic Sci Med Pathol* 2008;**4**:205–211.

Jung S, Kim M, Kim S et al. Interaction between γ-hydroxybutyric acid and ethanol: a review from toxicokinetic and toxicdynamic perspectives. *Metabolites* 2023;**13**:180.

Neu P, Danker-Hopfe H, Fisher R, Ehlen F. GHB: a life-threatening drug – complications and outcome of GHB detoxification treatment – an observational clinical study. *Addict Sci Clin Pract* 2023 Oct 21;**18**(1):62. doi: 10.1186/s13722-023-00414-w.

Scott-Ham M, Burton FC. Toxicological findings in cases of alleged drug-facilitated sexual assault in the United Kingdom over a 3-year period. *J Clin Forensic Med* 2005;**12**:175–186.

Tay E, Lo WKW, Murnion B. Current insights on the impact of gamma-hydroxybutyrate (GHB) abuse. *Subst Abuse & Rehab.* 2022;**13**:13–23.

Zvosec DL, Smith SW, Porrata T, et al. Case series of 226 γ-hydroxybutyrate-associated deaths: lethal toxicity and trauma. *Am J Emerg Med* 2011;**29**:319–332.

Ketamine

Burch HJ, Clarke EJ, Hubbard AM, et al. Concentrations of drugs determined in blood samples collected from suspected drugged drivers in England and Wales. *J Forensic Legal Med* 2013;**20**:278–289.

Cheng WC, Ng KM, Chan KK, Mok VKK, Cheung BKL. Roadside detection of impairment under the influence of ketamine – evaluation of ketamine impairment symptoms with reference to its concentration in oral fluid and urine. *Forensic Sci Int* 2007;**170**:51–58.

Corazza O, Schifano F, Simonato P, et al. Phenomenon of new drugs on the internet: the case of ketamine derivative methoxetamine. *Hum Psychopharmacol* 2012;**27**:145–149.

Dijkstra FM, ven der LOO AJAE, Abdulahad S et al. The effects of intranasal esketamine on onroad driving performance in patients with major depressive disorder or persistent depressive disorder. *J Psychopharmacol* 2022;**36**:614–625.

Edinoff AN, Sall, S, Koontz CB et al. Ketamine evolving clinical roles and potential effects with cognitive, motor and driving ability. *Neurol Int* 2023;**15**:352–361.

Hansen G, Jensen SB, Chandresh L, et al. The psychotropic effect of ketamine. *J Psychoactive Drugs* 1988;**20**:419–425.

Hofer KE, Grager B, Muller DM, et al. Ketamine-like effects after recreational use of methoxetamine. *Ann Emerg Med* 2012;**60**:97–99.

Jansen KLR. Non-medical use of ketamine. *BMJ* 1993;**306**:601–602.

Kohtala S. Ketamine—50 years in use: from anesthesia to rapid antidepressant effects and neurobiological mechanisms. *Pharmacol Reports* 2021;**73**;323–345.

Lucuta L, Maas-Gramlich A, Kraemer M, Andresen-Streichert H, Juebner M. Ketamine in DUID cases in the greater Cologne area. *Forensic Sci Int* 2024 Jan;**354**:111905. doi: 10.1016/j.forsciint.2023.111905. Epub 2023 Dec 5.

Mozayani A. Ketamine – effects on human performance and behaviour. *Forensic Sci Rev* 2002;**14**:123–131.

Pelletier R, Le Dare B, Le Bouedec D et al. Arylcyclohexylamine Derivatives: Pharmacokinetic, Pharmacodynamic, Clinical and Forensic Aspects. *Int J Mol Sci* 2022;**23**:15574.

Savić Vujović K, Jotić A, Medić B, Srebro D, Vujović A, Žujović J, Opanković A, Vučković S. Ketamine, an old-new drug: uses and abuses. *Pharmaceuticals (Basel)* 2023 Dec 21;**17**(1):16. doi: 10.3390/ph17010016.

Shields JE, Dargan PI, Wood DM, et al. Methoxetamine-associated reversible cerebellar toxicity: three cases with analytical confirmation. *Clin Toxicol* 2012;**50**:438–440.

Weiner AL, Viera L, McKay CA, Bayer MJ. Ketamine abusers presenting to the emergency department: a case series. *J Emerg Med* 2000;**18**: 447–451.

White PF, Way WL, Trevor AJ. Ketamine – its pharmacology and therapeutic uses. *Anesthesiology* 1982;**56**:119–136.

Winstock AR, Mitcheson L, Gillatt DA, Cottrell AM. The prevalence and natural history of urinary symptoms among recreational ketamine users. *BJU Int* 2012;**110**:1762–1766.

Wolff K, Winstock AR. Ketamine – from medicine to misuse. *CNS Drugs* 2006;**20**:199–218.

Wood DM, Davies S, Puchnarewicz M, et al. Acute toxicity associated with the recreational use of the ketamine derivative methoxetamine. *Eur J Clin Pharmacol* 2012;**68**:853–856.

Khat

Al-Maweri SA, Warnakulasuriya S, Samran A. Khat (Catha edulis) and its oral health effects: An updated review. J Investig Clin Dent. 2018 Feb;**9**(1). doi: 10.1111/jicd.12288.

Chappell JS, Lee MM. Cathinone preservation in khat evidence via drying. *Forensic Sci Int* 2010;**195**:108–120.

Corkery JM, Schifano F, Oyefeso A, et al. Overview of literature and information on 'khat-related' mortality: a call for recognition of the issue and further research. *Ann 1st Super Sanita* 2011;**47**:445–464.

Feigin A, Higgs P, Hellard M, Dietze P. Further research required to determine link between khat consumption and driver impairment. *Bull World Health Organ* 2010;**88**:480.

Giannini AJ, Castellani SJ. A manic-like psychosis due to khat. *J Toxicol Clin Toxicol* 1982;**19**:455–459.

Nencini P, Ahmed AM, Elmi AS. Subjective effects of khat chewing in humans. *Drug Alcohol Depend* 1985;**18**:97–105.

Silva B, Soares J, Rocha-Pereira C et al Khat, a cultural chewing drug: a toxicokinetic and toxicodynamic summary. *Toxins* 2022;**14**;71.

Toennes SW, Kauert GF. Driving under the influence of khat – alkaloid concentrations and observations in forensic cases. *Forensic Sci Int* 2004;**140**:85–90.

LSD

Gruman C, Henkel K, Brandt SD et al. Pharmacokinetics and subjective effects of 1P-LSD in humans after oral and intravenous administration. *Drug Testing & Anal* 2020;**12**:1144–1153.

Hofmann A., 1975. The chemistry of LSD and its modifications. In: *LSD A Total Study*. Westbury, NY:PED Publications.

Holze F, Liechti ME, Hutten NRPW et al. Pharmacokinetics and pharmacodynamics of lysergic acid diethylamide microdoses in healthy participants. *Clin Pharmacol & Therap* 2021;**109**:658–666.

Knudsen GM. Sustained effects of single doses of classical psychedelics in humans. *Neuropsychopharmacol* 2023;**48**:145–150.

Passie T, Halpern JH, Stichtinoth DO, et al. The pharmacology of lysergic acid diethylamide: a review. *CNS Neurosci Ther* 2008;**14**:295–314.

Paul BD, Smith ML. LSD – an overview on drug action and detection. *Forensic Sci Rev* 1999;**11**:157–174.

Ramaekers JG, Hutten N, Mason NL et al. *J Psychopharmacol* 2021;**35**:398–405.

Smart RG, Bateman K. Unfavourable reactions to LSD: a review and analysis of the available case reports. *Can Med Assoc J* 1967;**97**:1214–1221.

Smith DE, Seymour RB. Dream becomes nightmare. Adverse reactions to LSD. *J Psych Drugs* 1985;**17**:297–303.

Nitrites

Advisory Council on the Misuse of Drugs, 8 May 2024. *Alkyl Nitrites ("Poppers") – Updated Harms Assessment and Consideration of Exemption from the Psychoactive Substances Act (2016)*. https://www.gov.uk/government/publications/alkyl-nitrites-acmd-exemption-consideration (accessed 31 July 2024).

Bartolo C, Koklanis K, Vukicevic M. 'Poppers Maculopathy' and the adverse ophthalmic outcomes from the recreational use of alkyl nitrate inhalants: a systematic review. *Semin Ophthalmol* 2023 May;**38**(4):371–379. doi: 10.1080/08820538.2022.2108717.

Belzer A, Krasowski MD. Causes of acquired methemoglobinemia – a retrospective study at a large academic hospital. *Toxicol Rep* 2024 Mar 16;**12**: 331–337. doi: 10.1016/j.toxrep.2024.03.004.

Chiang C, Gessner N, Burli A et al. Poppers dermatitis®: a systematic review on a unique form of contact dermatitis® in the MSM community. *Dermatitis* 2024 May–Jun;**35**(3):198–204. doi: 10.1089/derm.2023.0157.

Gooley B, Lofy T, Gross J, Sonnenberg T, Feldman R. Ventricular fibrillation in a 21-year-old after inhalation of an isobutyl nitrite 'popper' product. *Am J Emerg Med.* 2023 Feb;**64**:204.e5–204.e7. doi: 10.1016/j. ajem.2022.10.048.

Haverkos HW, Kopstein AN, Wilson H, and Drotman P. Nitrite inhalants: history, epidemiology, and possible links to AIDS. *Environmental Health Perspectives* 1994;102: 858–861.

Kubic A, Wahl M., 2024 Amyl nitrite. *Encyclopedia of Toxicology* (fourth edition) Volume 1. Elsevier, pages 435–438.

Lowry TP. Psychosexual aspects of the volatile nitrites. *J Psychoactive Drugs* 1982 Jan–Jun;**14**(1–2):77–79. doi: 10.1080/02791072.1982.10471914.

Modarai B, Kapadia YK, Terris J. Methylene blue: a treatment for severe methaemoglobinaemia secondary to misuse of amyl nitrite. *Emerg Med J* 2002;19:270–271.

Movio G, Erskine K, Scullion S. Methaemoglobinaemia due to alkyl nitrites in a patient with suspected traumatic injuries. *BMJ Case Rep* 2023 May 29;16(5):e255131. doi: 10.1136/bcr-2023-255131.

Romanelli F, Smith KM, Thornton AC, Pomeroy C. Poppers: epidemiology and clinical management of inhaled nitrite abuse. *Pharmacotherapy* 2004;**24**:69–78.

Schwartz C, Tooley L, Knight R, Steinberg M. Queering poppers literature: a critical interpretive synthesis of health sciences research on alkyl nitrite use and Canadian policy. *International Journal of Drug Policy* 2022;**101**:103546.

Vaccher SJ, Hammoud MA, Bourne A, Lea T, Haire BG, Holt M, Saxton P, Mackie B, Badge J, Jin F, Maher L, Prestage G. Prevalence, frequency, and motivations for alkyl nitrite use among gay, bisexual and other men who have sex with men in Australia. *Int J Drug Policy* 2020 Feb;**76**:102659. doi: 10.1016/j.drugpo.2019.102659.

PMID: 31927224

Williams JF, Storck M, Committee on Substance Abuse, Committee on Native American Child Health. Inhalant abuse. *Pediatrics* 2007;**119**: 1009–1017.

Nitrous Oxide

Brunt TM, van den Brink W, van Amsterdam J. Mechanisms involved in the neurotoxicity and abuse liability of nitrous oxide: a narrative review. *Int J Mol Sci* 2022 Dec;**23**(23):14747. doi: 10.3390/ijms232 314747.

Davidson LT. Recreational use of nitrous oxide causes seizure, pneumothorax, pneumomediastinum, and pneumopericardium: nitrous oxide and its harm, a case report. *Ups J Med Sci* 2023 Dec 8:128. doi: 10.48101/ujms. v128.10281.

Fortanier E, Delmont E, Corazza G et al. Longitudinal follow-up and prognostic factors in nitrous oxide-induced neuropathy. *J Peripher Nerv Syst* 2024 Jun;**29**(2):252–261. doi: 10.1111/jns.12634.

Home Office, 2023. *Nitrous Oxide Ban: Guidance*. Crown copyright.

Patel SG, Zhang T, Liem B et al. Nitrous oxide myelopathy: a case series. *N Z Med J* 2024 Jul 19;**137**(1599):49–54. doi: 10.26635/6965.6477.

Paris A, Lake L, Joseph A et al. Nitrous oxide-induced subacute combined degeneration of the cord: diagnosis and treatment. *Pract Neurol* 2023 Jun;**23**(3):222–228. doi: 10.1136/pn-2022–003631.

Stone MJ, Roberts NM, Anwar MU. Burn injury from filling balloons with nitrous oxide. *BMJ Case Rep* 2021 Dec 1;**14**(12):e247077. doi: 10.1136/ bcr-2021–247077.

Verboeket SO, van den Bergh J, van Amsterdam J et al. Treatment seeking nitrous oxide users in addiction care: a comparison with cocaine users on clinical and treatment characteristics. *Eur Addict Res.* 2024 Jul 12:1–10. doi: 10.1159/000539860.

Opiates/Opioids

Bachs LC, Engeland A, Morland JG, Skirtveit S. The risk of motor vehicle accidents involving drivers with prescriptions for codeine or tramadol. *Clin Pharmacol Ther* 2009;**85**:596–599.

Burns RH, Pierre CM, Marathe JG, Ruiz-Mercado G, Taylor JL, Kimmel SD, Johnson SL, Fukuda HD, Assoumou SA. Partnering with state health departments to address injection-related infections during the opioid epidemic: experience at a safety net hospital. *Open Forum Infect Dis* 2021 Apr 27;**8**(8):ofab208. doi: 10.1093/ofid/ ofab208.

Darke S, Duflou J, Torok M. The comparative toxicology and major organ pathology of fatal methadone and heroin toxicity cases. *Drug Alcohol Depend* 2010;**106**:1–6.

Darke S, Zador D. Fatal heroin 'overdose': a review. *Addiction* 1996;**91**: 1765–1772.

Duhart Clark SE, Kral AH, Zibbell JE. Consuming illicit opioids during a drug overdose epidemic: illicit fentanyls, drug discernment, and the radical transformation of the illicit opioid market. *Int J Drug Policy* 2022;**99**:103467.

Glare PA, Walsh TD. Clinical pharmacokinetics of morphine. *Ther Drug Monitor* 1991;**13**:1–23.

Gordon NB, Appel PW. Functional potential of the methadone-maintained person. *Alcohol Drugs Driv* 1995;**11**:31–37.

Malcolm NJ, Palkovic B, Sprague DJ, Calkins MM et al. Mu-opioid receptor selective superagonists produce prolonged respiratory depression. *iScience* 2023;**26**:107121.

NICE Evidence review. Opioid dependence: buprenorphine prolonged release injection (Buvidal), February 2019 https://www.nice.org.uk/advice/es19/resources/opioid-dependence-buprenorphine-prolongedrelease-injection-buvidal-pdf-1158123740101.

Osborne R, Joel S, Trew D, Slevin M. Morphine and metabolite behavior after different routes of morphine administration: demonstration of the importance of the active metabolite morphine-6-glucuronide. *Clin. Pharmacol Ther* 1990;**47**:12–19.

Pergolizzi Jr J, Raffa R, LeQuang J K, et al. Old drugs and new challenges: a narrative review of nitazenes. *Cureus* 2023 June 21;**15**(6): e40736. doi:10.7759/cureus.40736.

Pirnay S, Borron SW, Giudicelli CP, Tourneau J, Baud FJ, Ricordel I. A critical review of the causes of death among post-mortem toxicological investigations: analysis of 34 buprenorphine-associated and 35 methadone-associated deaths. *Addiction* 2004;**99**:978–988.

Polettini A, Groppi A, Monagna M. The role of alcohol abuse in the etiology of heroin-related deaths. Evidence for pharmacokinetic interactions between heroin and alcohol. *J Analyt Toxicol* 1999;**23**:570–576.

Schindler S, Ortner R, Peternell A, et al. Maintenance therapy with synthetic opioids and driving aptitude. *Eur Addict Res* 2004;**10**:80–87.

Shafi A, Berry AJ, Sumnall H, Wood DM, Tracy DK. Synthetic opioids: a review and clinical update *Ther Adv Psychopharmacol* 2022;**12**:1–16.

Sporer KA. Acute heroin overdose. *Ann Intern Med* 1999;**130**:584–590.

Stout PR. Farrell LJ. Opioids – effects on human performance and behaviour. *Forensic Sci Rev* 2003; **15**:29–59.

Thiblin I, Eksborg S, Petersson A, Fugelstad A, Rajs J. Fatal intoxication as a consequence of intranasal administration (snorting) or pulmonary inhalation (smoking) of heroin. *Forensic Sci Int* 2004;**139**:241–247.

UNODC, March 2017. Global SMART Update Volume 17. UNODC.

Vandeputte, M., Van Uytfanghe, K., Layle, N., St Germaine, et al. Synthesis, chemical characterization, and mu-opioid receptor activity assessment of the emerging group of 'nitazene' 2-benzylbenzimidazole synthetic opioids. *ACS Chemical Neuroscience* 2021;**12** :1241–1251.

Vieweg WVR, Lipps WFC, Fernandez A, et al. Opioids and methadone equivalents for clinicians. *J Clin Psychiatry* 2005;7:86–88.

Walter LA, Bunnell S, Wiesendanger K, McGregor AJ. Sex, gender, and the opioid epidemic: crucial implications for acute care. *AEM Educ Train* 2022 Jun 23;6(Suppl 1):S64–S70. doi: 10.1002/aet2.10756.

Zacny JP. A review of the effects of opiates on psychomotor and cognitive functioning in humans. *Exp Clin Psychopharmacol* 1995;3:432–466.

Phencyclidine

Clardy DO, Gravey RH, MacDonald BJ, Wiersma SJ, Pearce, DS, Ragle JL. The phencyclidine-intoxicated driver. *Journal of Analytical Toxicology* 1979 Nov-Dec:3(6):238–241. https://doi.org/10.1093/jat/3.6.238.

Clouet DH, ed., 1986. NIDA Research Monograph 64: Phencyclidine – an update. Department of Health and Human Services, Public Health Service, Alcohol, Drug Abuse, and Mental Health Administration. https://archive.org/stream/bweiner_hazeldenbettyford_64/64_djvu.txt (accessed 31 July 2024).

Edinoff AN, Sall S, Koontz CB et al. Ketamine evolving clinical roles and potential effects with cognitive, motor and driving ability. *Neurol Int* 2023 Mar 3;15(1):352–361. doi:.3390/neurolint15010023.

Kunsman GW, Levine B, Costantino A, Smith ML. Phencyclidine blood concentrations in DRE cases. *J Analyt Toxicol* 1997;21:498–502.

Lodge D, Mercier MS. Ketamine and phencyclidine: the good, the bad and the unexpected. *Br J Pharmacol.* 2015 Sep;172(17):4254–4276. doi: 10.1111/bph.13222.

McCarron MM, Schulze BW, Thompson GA, Conder MC, Goetz WA. Acute phencyclidine intoxication: incidence of clinical findings in 1,000 cases. *Ann Emerg Med* 1981;10:237–242.

MacNeal JJ, Cone DC, Sinha V, et al. Use of haloperidol in PCP-intoxicated individuals. *Clin Toxicol* 2012;50:851–853.

Wiegand TJ., 2024. Phencyclidine. *Encyclopedia of Toxicology* (fourth edition). Elsevier, pages 515–519.

Phenethylamines

Acuna-Castillo A, Villalobos C, Moya PR, et al. Differences in potency and efficacy of a series of phenylisopropylamine/phenylethylamine pairs at 5-HT(2A) and 5-HT(2C) receptors. *Br J Pharmacol* 2002;136: 510–519.

de Boer D, Gijzels MJ, Bosman IJ, Maes RA. More data about the new psychoactive drug 2C-B. *J Analyt Toxicol* 1999;23:227–228.

Huang, HH, Bai, YM. Persistent psychosis after ingestion of a single tablet of '2C-B', *Progress in Neuro-Psychopharmacology & Biological Psychiatry* 2010;**35**(1):293–294.

McGrane O, Simmons J, Jacobsen E, Skinner C. Alarming trends in a novel class of designer drugs. *J Clin Toxicol* 2011;**1**(2).

Ng PC, Banerji S, Graham J et al. Adolescent exposures to traditional and novel psychoactive drugs, reported to National Poison Data System (NPDS), 2007–2017. Drug and Alcohol Dependence 2019;**202**:1–5.

Palamar JJ, Acosta P. A qualitative descriptive analysis of effects of psychedelic phenethylamines and tryptamines. *Hum Psychopharmacol* 2020 Jan;**35**(1):e2719. doi: 10.1002/hup.2719

Sacks J, Ray MJ, Williams S, et al. Fatal toxic leukoencephalopathy secondary to overdose of a new psychoactive designer drug 2C-E ('Europa'). *Proc (Bayl Med Cent)* 2012;**25**:374–376.

Shulgin AT, Shulgin A., 1991. *PiHKAL – A Chemical Love Story*. Berkeley, CA: Transform Press.

UNODC Laboratory and Scientific Service Portals. Phenylethylamines. https://www.unodc.org/LSS/SubstanceGroup/Details/275dd468-75a3-4609-9e96-cc5a2f0da467 (accessed 31 July 2024).

Villalbos CA, Bull P, Saez P, et al. 4-Bromo-2,5-dimethoxyphenethylamine (2C-B) and structurally related phenylethylamines are potent 5-HT2A receptor antagonists in *Xenopus laevis* oocytes. *Br J Pharmacol* 2004;**141**:1167–1174.

Wadowski PP, Giurgea GA, Schlager O, Luf A, Gremmel T, Hobl EL, Unterhumer S, Löffler-Stastka H, Koppensteiner R. Acute limb ischemia after intake of the phenylethylamine derivate NBOMe. *Int J Environ Res Public Health* 2019 Dec 12;**16**(24):5071. doi: 10.3390/ijerph16245071.

Wood DM, Looker JJ, Shaikh L, et al. Delayed onset of seizures and toxicity associated with recreational use of bromo-dragonfly. *J Med Toxicol* 2009;**5**:226–229.

Zuba D, Sekula K, Buczek A. 25C-NBOMe – new potent hallucinogenic substance identified on the drug market. *Forensic Sci Int* 2013;**227**:7–14.

Piperazines

Antia U, Lee HS, Kydd RR, Tingle MD, Russell BR. Pharmacokinetics of 'party pill' drug N-benzylpiperazine (BZP) in healthy human participants. *Forensic Sci Int* 2009;**186**:63–67.

Arbo MD, Bastos ML. Piperazine compounds as drugs of abuse. *Drug and Alcohol Dependence* 2012;**122**(3):174–185.

Elliott S. Current awareness of piperazines: pharmacology and toxicology. *Drug Test Anal* 2011;**3**:430–438.

Elliott S, Smith C. Investigation of the first deaths in the United Kingdom involving detection and quantitation of the piperazines BZP and 3-TFMPP. *J Analyt Toxicol* 2008;**32**:172–177.

Gee P, Gilbert M, Richardson S, Moore G, Paterson S, Graham P. Toxicity from the recreational use of 1-benylpiperazine. *Clin Toxicol* 2008;**46**:802–807.

Gee, P, Jerram T, Bowie D. Multiorgan failure from 1-benzylpiperazine ingestion–legal high or lethal high? *Clinical Toxicology* 2010;**48**:230–233.

Gee P, Richardson S, Woltersdorg W, Moore G. Toxic effects of BZP-based herbal party pills in humans: a prospective study in Christchurch, New Zealand. *N Z Med J* 2005 Dec 16;**118**(1227):U1784.

Lin JC, Jan RK, Kydd RR, Russell BR. Subjective effects in human following administration of party pill drugs BZP and TFMPP alone and in combination. *Drug Test Anal* 2011;**3**:582–585.

Schep LJ, Slaughter RJ, Vale A, Beasley M, Gee GP. The clinical toxicology of the designer 'party pills' benzylpiperazine and trifluoromethylphenylpiperazine. *Clin Toxicol* 2011;**49**:131–141.

Sheridan J, Butler R, Wilkins C, Russell B. Legal piperazines-containing party pills – a new trend in substance misuse. *Drug Alcohol Rev* 2007;**26**:335–343.

Tancer ME, Johanson CE. The subjective effects of MDMA and mCPP in moderate MDMA users. *Drug Alcohol Depend* 2001;**65**:97–101.

Thompson I, William G, Caldwell B, et al. Randomised double-blind, placebo-controlled trial of the effects of the 'party pills' BZP/TFMPP alone and in combination with alcohol. *J Psychopharmacol* 2010;**24**:1299–1308.

UNODC Early Warning Advisory on New Psychoactive Substances. Piperazines. https://www.unodc.org/LSS/SubstanceGroup/Details/8242b801-355c-4454-9fdc-ba4b7e7689d5 (accessed 31 July 2024).

Welz A, Koba M, Kośliński P, Siódmiak J. Comparison of LC-MS and LC-DAD Methods of detecting abused piperazine designer drugs. *J Clin Med* 2022 Apr;**11**(7):1758. doi: 10.3390/jcm11071758.

Pipradrols

Coppola M, Mondola R. Research chemicals marketed as legal highs: the case of pipradrol derivatives. *Toxicology Letters* 2012;**1**: 57–60.

Iversen L, White M, Treble R. Designer psychostimulants: pharmacology and differences. *Neuropharmacology* 2014 Jan 15. doi: 10.1016/j.neuropharm.2014.01.015.

Kriikku P, Wilhelm L, Rintatalo J et al. Prevalence and blood concentrations of desoxypipradol (2-DPMP) in drivers suspected of driving under the influence of drugs and in post-mortem cases. *Forensic Sci Int* 2013;**226**: 146–151.

Lidder S, Dargan P, Sexton M et al. Cardiovascular toxicity associated with recreational use of diphenylprolinol (diphenyl-2-pyrrolidinemethanol [D2PM]). *J Med Toxicol* 2008;**4**:167–169.

Loi B, Sahai MA, De Luca MA, Shiref H, Opacka-Juffry J. The role of dopamine in the stimulant characteristics of novel psychoactive substances (NPS) – neurobiological and computational assessment using the case of desoxypipradrol (2-DPMP). *Front Pharmacol* 2020 Jun 5;**11**:806. doi: 10.3389/fphar.2020.00806.

Murray DB, Potts S, Haxton C et al. 'Ivory wave' toxicity in recreational drug users; integration of clinical and poisons information services to manage legal high poisoning. *Clin Toxicol (Phila)* 2012 Feb;**50**(2):108–113. doi: 10.3109/15563650.2011.647992.

Simmler LD, Rickli A, Schramm Y et al. Pharmacological profiles of aminoindanes, piperazines and pipradrol derivatives. *Biochem Pharmacol* 2014;**88**:237–244.

White MW, Archer JRH., 2013. Pipradrol and pipradrol derivatives. In: *Novel Psychoactive Substances Classification, Pharmacology and Toxicology.* Academic Press, pages 233–259.

Wood DM, Dargan PI. Use and acute toxicity associated with the novel psychoactive substances diphenylprolinol (D2PM) and desoxypipradrol (2-DPMP). *Clin Toxicol* 2012;**50**:727–732.

Synthetic Cannabinoids

Alzu'bi A, Almahasneh F, Khasawneh R et al. The synthetic cannabinoids menace: a review of health risks and toxicity. *Eur J Med Res* 2024 Jan 12;**29**(1):49. doi: 10.1186/s40001-023-01443-6.

Armstrong F, McCurdy MT, Heavner MS. Synthetic cannabinoid-associated multiple organ failure: case series and literature review. *Pharmacotherapy J Human Pharmacol Drug Therapy* 2019;**39**:508–513. doi: 10.1002/phar.2241.

Atwood BK, Lee D, Straiker A, et al. CP47, 497-C8 and JWH-073, commonly found in 'spice' herbal blends, are potent and efficacious CB1 cannabinoid receptor agonists. *Eur J Pharmacol* 2011;**659**:139–145.

Editorial. Turning down the spice: tackling the problems of synthetic cannabinoids. *BMJ* 2023 August 21;**382**. doi: https://doi.org/10.1136/bmj-2023-076611.

Ergelen M, Yalçın M, Bilici R. The comparison of violence, and the relationship with childhood trauma in Turkish men with alcohol, opiate, and synthetic cannabinoid use disorder. *Neuropsychiatr Dis Treat* 2018 Nov 23;**14**: 3169–3178. doi: 10.2147/NDT.S173604.

Gunderson EW, Haughey HM, Ait-Daoud N, et al. 'Spice' and 'K2' herbal highs: a case series and systematic review of the clinical effects and biopsychosocial implications of synthetic cannabinoid use in humans. *Am J Addict* 2012;21:320–326.

Hamzekalayi MRH, Ardakani MH, Moeini Z et al. A systematic review of novel cannabinoids and their targets: insights into the significance of structure in activity. *Eur J Pharmacol* 2024 Aug 5;976:176679. doi: 10.1016/j.ejphar.2024.176679.

Harris CR, Brown A. Synthetic cannabinoid intoxication: A case series and review. *J Emerg Med* 2013;44:360–366.

Heal DJ, Gosden J, Smith SL. A critical assessment of the abuse, dependence and associated safety risks of naturally occurring and synthetic cannabinoids. *Front Psychiatry* 2024 Jun 10;15:1322434. doi: 10.3389/fpsyt.2024.1322434.

Hermanns-Clausen M, Kneisel S, Szabo B, et al. Acute toxicity due to the confirmed consumption of synthetic cannabinoids: clinical and laboratory findings. *Addiction* 2013;108:534–544.

Humayun M, Suarez JI, Shah VA. Neurological Complications of Cannabinoids. *Semin Neurol* 2024 Aug;44(4):430–440. doi: 10.1055/s-0044–1787570.

Maglaviceanu A, Peer M, Rockel J et al. The state of synthetic cannabinoid medications for the treatment of pain. *CNS Drugs* 2024 Aug;38(8):597–612. doi: 10.1007/s40263-024-01098-9.

Mushoff F, Madea B, Kernbach-Wighton G, et al. Driving under the influence of synthetic cannabinoids ('spice'): a case series. *Int J Legal Med* 2014;128:59–64.

Orazietti V, Basile G, Giorgetti R, Giorgetti A. Effects of synthetic cannabinoids on psychomotor, sensory and cognitive functions relevant for safe driving. *Front Psychiatry* 2022 Sep 26;13:998828. doi: 10.3389/fpsyt.2022.998828.

Rajasekaran M, Brents LK, Franks LN, et al. Human metabolites of synthetic cannabinoids JWH-018 and JWH-073 bind with high affinity and act as potent agonists at cannabinoid type-2 receptors. *Toxicol Appl Pharmacol* 2013;269:100–108.

Sheikh IA, Lukšič M, Ferstenberg R, Culpepper-Morgan JA. Spice/K2 synthetic marijuana-induced toxic hepatitis treated with N-acetylcysteine. *Am J Case Rep* 2014;15:584–588. doi: 10.12659/AJCR.891399.

Synthetic Cathinones

Baumann MH, Partilla JS, Lehner KR. Psychoactive 'bath salts': not so soothing. *Eur J Pharmacol* 2013;698:1–5.

Burch HJ, Clarke EJ, Hubbard AM, et al. Concentrations of drugs determined in blood samples collected from suspected drugged drivers in England and Wales. *J Forensic Legal Med* 2013;**20**:278–289.

Chen S, Zhou W, Lai M. Synthetic cathinones: epidemiology, toxicity, potential for abuse, and current public health perspective. *Brain Sci* 2024 Mar 29;**14**(4):334. doi: 10.3390/brainsci14040334.

Corkery J, Schifano F, Ghodse AH, et al., 2012. Mephedrone-related fatalities in the United Kingdom. In: Gallelli L (ed.), *Contextual, Clinical and Practical Issues. Pharmacology*. InTech.

Cosbey SH, Peters KL, Quinn A, et al. Mephedrone (Methylmethcathinone) in toxicology casework: a Northern Ireland perspective. *J Analyt Toxicol* 2013;**37**:74–82.

Dargan PI, Sedefov R, Gallegos A, et al. The pharmacology and toxicology of the synthetic cathinone mephedrone (4-methylmethcathinone). *Drug Test Anal* 2011;**3**:454–463.

Daswani RR, Choles CM, Kim DD, Barr AM. A systematic review and meta-analysis of synthetic cathinone use and psychosis. *Psychopharmacology (Berl)* 2024 May;**241**(5):875–896. doi: 10.1007/s00213-024-06569-x.

Daziani G, Lo Faro AF, Montana V et al. Synthetic cathinones and neurotoxicity risks: a systematic review. *Int J Mol Sci* 2023 Mar 25;**24**(7):6230. doi: 10.3390/ijms24076230.

De Felice LJ, Glennon RA, Negus SS. Synthetic cathinones: chemical phylogeny, physiology and neuropharmacology. *Life Sci* 2014;**97**:20–26.

EMCDDA Risk Assessments, 2011. *Report on the Risk-assessments of Mephedrone in the Framework of the Council Decision on New Psychoactive Drugs*, No. 9. Lisbon: EMCDDA.

Kelly JP. Cathinone derivatives: a review of their chemistry, pharmacology and toxicology. *Drug Test Anal* 2011;**3**:439–453.

Maas A, Wippich C, Madea B, Hess C. Driving under the influence of synthetic phenethylamines: a case series. *Int J Legal Med* 2015 Sep;**129**(5):997–1003. doi: 10.1007/s00414-015-1150-1.

Maskell PD, De Paoli G, Seneviratne C, et al. Mephedrone (4-methylmethcathinone)-related deaths. *J Analyt Toxicol* 2011;**35**:189–191.

Miotto K, Striebel J, Cho AK et al. Clinical and pharmacological aspects of bath salt use: a review of the literature and case reports. *Drug & Alc Depend* 2013;**132**:1–12.

Pieprzyca E, Skowronek R, Czekaj P. Toxicological analysis of cases of mixed poisonings with synthetic cathinones and other drugs of abuse. *J Anal Toxicol* 2023 Jan 24;**46**(9):1008–1015. doi: 10.1093/jat/bkab119.

Prosser JM, Nelson LS. The toxicology of bath salts: a review of synthetic cathinones. *J Med Toxicol* 2012;**8**:33–42.

Simmler LD, Rickli A, Hoener MC et al. Monoamine transporter and receptor interaction profiles of a new series of designer cathinones. *Neuropharmacol* 2014;79:152–160.

Warrick BJ, Wilson J, Hedge M, Freeman S, Leonard K, Aaron C. Lethal serotonin syndrome after methylone and butylone ingestion. *J Med Toxicol* 2012;8:65–68.

Tobacco

Alam N, Mariam W. Impact of tobacco habits on poor oral health status among bone-factory workers in a low literacy city in India: a cross-sectional study. *PLoS One* 2024 Apr 17;19(4):e0299594. doi: 10.1371/journal. pone.0299594.

Alamer NI, Alsaleh A, Alkhaldi S. Tobacco products and oral conditions among US adults: NHANES 2017–2020. *J Public Health Dent.* 2024 Jun;84(2):206–212. doi: 10.1111/jphd.12615.

Editorial. The rise of disposable e-cigarettes in England and implications for public health. BMJ 2024 July 17;386. doi: https://doi.org/10.1136/bmj. q1508.

López-Cervantes JP, Schlünssen V, Senaratna C et al. Use of oral moist tobacco (snus) in puberty and its association with asthma in the population-based RHINESSA study. *BMJ Open Respir Res* 2024 Jul 22;11(1):e002401. doi: 10.1136/bmjresp-2024–002401.

Kassem NOF, Strongin RM, Stroup AM et al. Toxicity of waterpipe tobacco smoking: the role of flavors, sweeteners, humectants, and charcoal. *Toxicol Sci* 2024 Jul 22:kfae095. doi: 10.1093/toxsci/kfae095.

Moylan S, Jacka FN, Pasco JA, Berk M. Cigarette smoking, nicotine dependence and anxiety disorders: a systematic review of population-based, epidemiological studies. *BMC Med* 2012;10:123.

Ondrejka J, Giorgio G. Type 1 Brugada pattern associated with nicotine toxicity. *J Emerg Med* 2015 Dec;49(6):e183–6. doi: 10.1016/j. jemermed.2015.08.008.

Shao XM, Fang ZT. Severe acute toxicity of inhaled nicotine and e-cigarettes: seizures and cardiac arrhythmia. *Chest.* 2020 Mar;157(3):506–508. doi: 10.1016/j.chest.2019.10.008.

Ueda K, Kawachi I, Nakamura M, et al. Cigarette nicotine yields and nicotine intake among Japanese male workers. *Tobacco Control* 2002;11:55–60.

Tuisku A, Rahkola M, Nieminen P, Toljamo T. Electronic cigarettes vs Varenicline for smoking cessation in adults: a randomized clinical trial. *JAMA Intern Med* 2024 Jun 17:e241822. doi: 10.1001/jamainternmed.2024.1822.

Vojjala M, Stevens ER, Nicholson A et al. Switching to e-cigarettes as harm reduction among individuals with chronic disease who currently smoke: results of a pilot randomized controlled trial. *Nicotine Tob Res* 2024 Jul 12:ntae158. doi: 10.1093/ntr/ntae158.

Weeks GR, Gobarani RK, Abramson MJ et al. Varenicline and nicotine replacement therapy for smokers admitted to hospitals: a randomized clinical trial. *JAMA Netw Open* 2024 Jun 3;7(6):e2418120. doi: 10.1001/jamanetworkopen.2024.18120.

Tryptamines

Barker SA, Monti JA, Christian ST, et al. *N, N*-Dimethyltryptamine – an endogenous hallucinogen. *Int Rev Neurobiol* 1981;**22**:83–110.

Bienemann B, Ruschel N, Campos ML et al. Self-reported negative outcomes of psilocybin users: a quantitative textual analysis. *PLoS One* 2020 Feb 21;**15**(2):e0229067. doi: 10.1371/journal.pone.0229067.

Boland DM, Andollo W, Hime GW, Hearn WL. Fatality due to acute alphamethyltryptamine intoxication. *J Anal Toxicol* 2005 Jul–Aug;**29**(5):394–397. doi: 10.1093/jat/29.5.394.

Chamakura RP. Bufotenine – a hallucinogen in ancient snuff powders of South America and a drug of abuse on the streets of New York City. *Forensic Sci Rev* 1994;**6**:1–18.

Corkery JM, Durkin E, Elliott S et al. The recreational tryptamine 5-MeO-DALT (N,N-diallyl-5-methoxytryptamine): a brief review. *Progr in Neuropsychopharmacol & Biol Psychiatry* 2011;**39**:259–262.

Hasler F, Grimberg U, Benz MA, Huber T, Vollenweider FX. Acute psychological and physiological effects of psilocybin in healthy humans: a double-blind, placebo-controlled dose-effect study. *Psychopharmacology* 2004;**172**:145–156.

Jovel A. Felthouse A, Bhattacharyya A. Delirium due to intoxication from the novel synthetic tryptamine. 5-MeO-Dalt. *Journal of Forensic Sciences* 2014;**59**(3):844–846.

King LA, Nutt DJ, Nichold DE. Remove barriers to clinical research for schedule 1 drugs with therapeutic potential. *BMJ* 2023 May 2;381. doi: https://doi.org/10.1136/bmj.p981.

Meatherall R, Sharma PJ. Foxy, a designer tryptamine hallucinogen. *J Analyt Toxicol* 2003;**27**:313–317.

Passie T, Seifert J, Schneider U, Emrich HM. The pharmacology of psilocybin. *Addict Biol* 2002;**7**:357–364.

Riba J, Valle M, Urbano G, et al. Human pharmacology of ayahuasca: subjective and cardiovascular effects, monoamine metabolite excretion and pharmacokinetics. *J Pharmacol Exp Ther* 2003;**306**:73–83.

Shulgin AT, Shulgin A., 1997. *TiHKAL: The Continuation*. Berkeley, CA: Transform Press.

Tiscione NB, Miller MI. Psilocin identified in a DUID investigation. *J Anal Toxicol* 2006 Jun;**30**(5):342–345. doi: 10.1093/jat/30.5.342.

UNODC Early Warning Advisory on New Psychoactive Substances. Tryptamine. UNODC. https://www.unodc.org/LSS/SubstanceGroup/Details/68c027b6-0ed9-4c07-a139-7f1ca7ffce84

Wright TH. Suspected driving under the influence case involving mitragynine. *Toxicol* 2018 Sep 1;**42**(7):e65–e68. doi: 10.1093/jat/bky028.

Volatile Substances

Butland BK, Field-Smith ME, Ramsey JD, et al. Twenty-five years of volatile substance abuse mortality: a national mortality surveillance programme. *Addiction* 2013;**108**:385–393.

Channer KS, Stanley S. Persistent visual hallucinations secondary to chronic solvent encephalopathy: case report and review of the literature. *J Neurol Neurosurg Psychiatry* 1983;**46**:83–86.

Flanagan RJ, Streete PJ, Ramsey JD., 1997. *Volatile Substance Abuse: Practical Guidelines for Analytical Investigation of Suspected Cases and Interpretation of Results*. UNDCP Technical Series No. 5. Vienna: United Nations Drug Control Programme.

Gunn J, Wilson J, Mackintosh AF. Butane sniffing causing ventricular fibrillation. *Lancet* 1989;**i**:617.

Kim J, Choe S, Shin I et al. Analytical methods for detecting butane, propane, and their metabolites in biological samples: implications for inhalant abuse detection. *J Chromatogr B Analyt Technol Biomed Life Sci* 2024 Feb 15:**1234**:124011. doi: 10.1016/j.jchromb.2024.124011.

King MD, Day RE, Oliver RS, et al. Solvent encephalopathy. *BMJ* 1981;**283**:663–665.

Piersanti V, Napoletano G, David MC. Sudden death due to butane abuse – an overview. *J Forensic Leg Med* 2024 Apr:**103**:102662. doi: 10.1016/j.jflm.2024.102662.

Roberts MJD, McIvor RA, Adgey AAJ. Asystole following butane gas inhalation. *Br J Hosp Med* 1990;**44**:294.

Schneider KE, Martin EM, Allen ST et al. Volatile drug use and overdose during the first year of the COVID-19 pandemic in the United States. *Int J Drug Policy* 2024 Apr;**126**:104371. doi: 10.1016/j.drugpo.2024. 104371.

Siegel E, Wason S. Sudden death caused by inhalation of butane and propane. *N Engl J Med* 1990;**323**:1638.

'Z' Drugs

Benavente R, Parada N, Sánchez B et al. Sulfhemoglobinemia secondary to the use of zopiclone. Report of two cases. [In Spanish] *Rev Med Chil* 2022 Oct;150(10):1401–1406. doi: 10.4067/S0034-9887202200 1001401.

Drover DR. Comparative pharmacokinetics and pharmacodynamics of short-acting hypnosedatives zaleplon, zolpidem and zopiclone. *Clin Pharmacokinet* 2004;**43**:227–238.

Garnier R, Guerault E, Muzard D, et al. Acute zolpidem poisoning – analysis of 344 cases. *Clin Toxicol* 1994;**32**:391–404.

Glancy M, Palmateer N, Yeung A et al. Risk of drug-related death associated with co-prescribing of gabapentinoids and Z-drugs among people receiving opioid-agonist treatment: a national retrospective cohort study. *Psychiatry Res.* 2024 Jun 12;**339**:116028. doi: 10.1016/j.psychres.2024. 116028.

Greenblatt DJ, Zammit GK. Pharmacokinetic evaluation of eszopiclone: clinical and therapeutic implications. *Expert Opin Drug Metab Toxicol* 2012 Dec;**8**(12):1609–1618. doi: 10.1517/17425255.2012. 741588.

Gunja N. In the zzz zone: the effects of z drugs on human performance and driving. *J Med Toxicol* 2013;**9**:163–171.

Lader M. Zopiclone: is there any dependence and abuse potential? *J Neurol* 1997;**244**(suppl 1):S18–22.

National Institute for Health & Care Excellence, 2023. Should I stop my benzodiazepine or z-drug? NICE.

Noble S, Langtry HD, Lamb HM. Zopiclone: an update of its pharmacology, clinical efficacy and tolerability in the treatment of insomnia. *Drugs* 1998;**55**:277–302.

Reith DM, Fountain J, McDowell R, Tilyard M. Comparison of the fatal toxicity index of zopiclone with benzodiazepines. *J Toxicol Clin Toxicol* 2003;**41**:975–980.

Terzano MG, Rossi M, Palomba V, et al. New drugs for insomnia: comparative tolerability of zopiclone, zolpidem, and zaleplon. *Drug Safety* 2003;26:261–282.

Zhou M, Liu R, Tang J, Tang S. Effects of new hypnotic drugs on cognition: A systematic review and network meta-analysis. *Sleep Med X* 2023 Nov 19;6:100094. doi: 10.1016/j.sleepx.2023.100094.

Zullo AR, Khan MA, Pfeiffer MR et al. Non-benzodiazepine Hypnotics and Police-Reported Motor Vehicle Crash Risk among Older Adults: A Sequential Target Trial Emulation. *Am J Epidemiol* 2024 Jul 2:kwae168. doi: 10.1093/aje/kwae168. Online ahead of print.

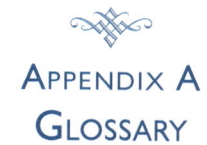

APPENDIX A
GLOSSARY

A selection of medical, technical and street terms in substance use. Many of the names of drugs are referred to within the main text under the specific drug.

The street terms for drugs expand and change with regularity – as with those terms mentioned in relation to specific drugs, the terms below are those accepted medically, or have had regular street usage.

Please note that spellings of certain drug names vary from country to country and anyone using this book should ensure that they are making reference to the appropriate drug and name within their jurisdiction.

Abstinence – the act of refraining from the use of a substance that may lead to withdrawal syndromes such as delirium tremens or barbiturate withdrawal

Acid – LSD

Acid head – LSD user

Adam – ecstasy (MDMA)

Addict – a person shall be regarded as being addicted to a drug if, and only if, he has as a result of repeated administration become so dependent upon the drug that he has an overpowering desire for the administration of it to be continued [The Misuse of Drugs Regulations 2001 (F95 (9)) https://www.legislation.gov.uk/uksi/2001/3998/2020-06-24]

ADME – refers to the processes of drug absorption (A), distribution (D), metabolism (M) and excretion (E)

Amp(s) – ampoule(s) of drugs

Angel dust – phencyclidine

Ataxia – disturbance of coordination of movement

Bag – small quantity of drugs

Barbs – barbiturate group of drugs, e.g. amylobarbital, phenobarbital

Bath salts – cathinone-type drugs

Benzos – benzodiazepine group of drugs, e.g. diazepam, nitrazepam

Billy whizz – amphetamines

Binge – heavy episodic use of drugs (frequently alcohol, cocaine and more recently synthetic cathinones)

Bioavailability – the percentage of the administered drug that arrives unchanged in the body circulation

Biological fluid – any fluid found in the body; may include saliva, sweat, blood or urine, or vitreous humour – all of which may be used to detect drug presence

Bolivian marching powder – cocaine

Bong – pipe for smoking cannabis

Brown – heroin

Buds – pregabalin

Catecholamine – a group of hormones including adrenaline, noradrenaline and dopamine, all involved as transmitter substances in the brain

Charlie – cocaine (generally as powder)

Chasing the dragon – smoking heroin off tinfoil

Clucking – withdrawing from drugs (generally opiates)

C_{max} – maximum concentration that a drug reaches in the circulation after a single dose

CNS – central nervous system

Coke – cocaine

Crack – freebase form of cocaine; can be smoked (names include, rock, white, base)

Crystal meth – methamphetamine

Detoxification – the process whereby drug withdrawal is managed in a person dependent on alcohol or other drugs

DIC – disseminated intravascular coagulation

Dopamine – transmitter substance in brain function – a catecholamine

Dose–response effect – the likelihood and severity of an effect of a drug related to the amount of exposure to the drug

Drug – any substance, other than those required for the maintenance of normal health, which, when taken into the living organism, may modify one or more of its functions (World Health Organization)

Drug dependence (also chemical or substance use disorder) see Chapter 1

Drug misuse – has been defined as any taking of a drug that harms or threatens to harm the physical and mental health or social wellbeing of an individual, other individuals or society at large, or that is illegal (Royal College of Psychiatrists, 1987)

Drug paraphernalia – items associated with drug use, e.g. syringes, needles, foil, citric acid, scales

DVLA – Driver and Vehicle Licensing Agency (in the UK)

Dysarthria – slurred speech – difficulty in articulation

E – ecstasy

ELISA – enzyme-linked immunosorbent assay – type of test used to identify drugs in biological fluids

First-pass metabolism – a process by which drugs are destroyed prior to entering the systemic circulation

Fix – injection of drugs

Flashbacks – spontaneous involuntary recurrences of drug-induced experiences

Foil – heroin may be smoked off tinfoil

Freebase – cocaine in its freebase form

Gabbies – gabapentin

Ganja – herbal cannabis

GBL – γ-butyrolactone

Gear – illegal drugs in general

GHB – γ-hydroxybutyrate

Grass – herbal cannabis

Habit (habituation) – having an addiction/dependence on a drug

Half-life – the time taken for the concentration of a drug in blood to reduce to half (assists in determining how long the effects of a drug will last)

Hippy crack – nitrous oxide

Horse tranquilliser – ketamine

Hyperpyrexia – raised temperature

Ice – crystalline form of methamphetamine

Immunoassay – a type of biochemical test for measuring amounts of substances in biological fluids

Intramuscular injection (IM) – injecting directly into a muscle

Intravenous injection (IV) – injecting a drug directly into a vein (mainlining)

Ivory wave – cathinone-type drugs including MDPV

Johnnies – gabapentin

Joint – hand-rolled cannabis cigarette

Khat – leaves of *Catha edulis*

Kratom – hallucinogenic substance derived from the plant Mitragyna speciosa

Laughing gas – nitrous oxide

Legal high – A substance with stimulant or mood-altering properties whose sale or use is not banned by current legislation regarding the misuse of drugs (see also NPS)

Linctus – methadone

Liquid ecstasy – γ-hydroxybutyrate

Liquid gold – amyl nitrite and related substances

Liquid X – γ-hydroxybutyrate

Magic mushrooms – hallucinogenic mushrooms e.g. psilocybin

Maintenance treatment – continued use of substitution treatment as an alternative to detoxification; may be required where an individual has relapsed on several occasions after detoxification

Marijuana – herbal (leaf) cannabis

M-Cat – cathinone-type drugs – often mephedrone or similar

MDMA – methylenedioxymethamphetamine (ecstasy)

Metabolite – breakdown product of the drug consumed

Meth – methamphetamine

Mexxy – methoxetamine

Miaow miaow – cathinone-type drugs – often mephedrone or similar

Microdots – LSD

Moggies – nitrazepam (Mogadon)

Molly – MDMA (and related compounds)

Moroccan – cannabis resin

Morphine (unconjugated morphine) – as morphine sulphate, its form after administration but before metabolism in the liver; becomes conjugated morphine in the liver, mainly morphine-3-glucuronide

Mule – someone who smuggles drugs, often internally (see 'stuffer')

Munchies – excess eating stimulated by (generally) cannabis

Mushies – hallucinogenic mushrooms

MXE – methoxetamine

N2O – nitrous oxide

Nabis – cannabis

Nasal insufflation – inhaling of substances into the body via the nose

New psychoactive substance (NPS) are drugs that are designed to replicate the effects of other illegal substances. People may refer to these drugs as 'legal highs', but all psychoactive substances are now either under the control of the Misuse of Drugs Act 1971 or subject to the Psychoactive Substances Act 2016 (PS Act).

Nitazenes – a group of synthetic drugs with powerful opiate-like effects

Nitro – amyl nitrite

Nox – nitrous oxide

NRG – cathinone-type drugs

Nystagmus – spontaneous rapid rhythmic eye movements in a side-to-side (horizontal) or up-and-down (vertical) direction

Opiates – drugs derived from the opium poppy e.g. codeine, morphine

Opioids – drugs with a treatment role in pain relief, by binding to brain opioid receptors which includes synthetic drugs e.g. methadone as well as opiates

Parenteral – generally, administration of a drug by an injection – via vein, artery, muscle or subcutaneous tissue

Pharmacodynamics – the effects of drugs on the body

Pharmacokinetics – the effects of the body on a drug

Plant food – cathinone-type drugs

Polydrug misuse – the use of more than one drug at the same time often used to titrate desired effects, ease comedown etc. Very commonly encountered; common combinations include opiates and benzodiazepines, stimulant drugs with cannabis and/or benzodiazepines. It is not uncommon to find an individual addicted to opiates and benzodiazepines

Poppers – amyl nitrite and related substances

Psychoactive – any substance that affects the central nervous system and affects behaviour

Puff – herbal cannabis

Qat – khat (leaves of *Catha edulis*)

Rattling – withdrawing from drugs (generally opiates)

Recreational use (of a drug) – the use of a drug intermittently for pleasure, not associated with dependence on that drug

Reefer – cannabis cigarette

Rehabilitation – restoration of normal function

Rizla – cigarette paper – often used to roll drugs with tobacco

Rock – freebase cocaine

Roid rage – extreme aggression and violence in association with steroid use

Roofies – Rohypnol tablets

RTC – road traffic collision (formerly known as RTA – road traffic accident)

Rush – an immediate sensation of wellbeing after taking a substance

Russian Valium – phenazepam

Salt water – γ-hydroxybutyrate

Sativa – herbal cannabis

Score – to buy drugs

Script – a prescription for a drug – commonly a heroin substitute such as methadone or buprenorphine

Skin pop – the practice of injecting drugs into tissue under the skin, often leaving circular depressed scars

Skunk – potent form of cannabis

Smack – heroin

Snort – inhale drugs up nose

Snow – cocaine powder

Special K – ketamine

Speed – amphetamine

Speedball – heroin and cocaine mixed and injected (also known as snowball)

Spice – synthetic cannabinoid compounds

Spliff – hand-rolled cannabis cigarette

Stack – use of oral and injected anabolic steroids in gym culture

Stash – concealed supply of drugs

Stereotypia – persistent repetition of words or movements

Stuffer – someone who conceals large quantities of drugs in body cavities (rectum, vagina, intestine), e.g. in condoms, for purposes of smuggling

Sulphate/sulph – amphetamines

Swallower – someone who has swallowed drugs – perhaps with the intention to conceal

Sweet air – nitrous oxide

Synaesthesia – the experience of 'hearing colours' and 'seeing sounds'

Tab – cigarette or LSD paper

Temazzy – temazepam tablets

THC – tetrahydrocannabinol – active ingredient of cannabis

Tolerance (to a drug) – the need to increase the drug dose to get the same effect or where the same dose of a drug produces a reduced effect – occurs after repeated use of certain drugs as the body adapts

Tony – a nitazene drug

Tracks – the line(s) (often discoloured like a bruise) along a vein where impure materials (most injectable illicit drugs) have been injected. May be evident for many days or weeks

Vitamin K – ketamine

Vitreous humour – the vitreous humour is the clear gel that fills the space between the lens and the retina of the eyeball of humans

Weed – cannabis

Withdrawal – the individual or cluster of symptoms and signs that are associated with the abstinence from longer-term use of some drugs (e.g. delirium tremens)

Works – needles and syringes used for injection

Wrap – small quantity of drugs

XTC – ecstasy

CLINICAL INSTITUTE WITHDRAWAL ASSESSMENT OF ALCOHOL SCALE, REVISED (CIWA-AR)

Patient: _____ **Date:** _____ **Time:** _____ (24 hour clock, midnight = 00:00)

Pulse or heart rate, taken for one minute: _____ **Blood pressure:** _____

NAUSEA AND VOMITING – Ask "Do you feel sick to your stomach? Have you vomited?" Observation.

0 no nausea and no vomiting
1 mild nausea with no vomiting
2
3
4 intermittent nausea with dry heaves
5
6
7 constant nausea, frequent dry heaves and vomiting

TACTILE DISTURBANCES – Ask "Have you any itching, pins and needles sensations, any burning, any numbness, or do you feel bugs crawling on or under your skin?" Observation.

0 none
1 very mild itching, pins and needles, burning or numbness
2 mild itching, pins and needles, burning or numbness
3 moderate itching, pins and needles, burning or numbness
4 moderately severe hallucinations
5 severe hallucinations
6 extremely severe hallucinations
7 continuous hallucinations

TREMOR – Arms extended and fingers spread apart. Observation.

0 no tremor
1 not visible, but can be felt fingertip to fingertip
2
3
4 moderate, with patient's arms extended
5
6
7 severe, even with arms not extended

AUDITORY DISTURBANCES – Ask "Are you more aware of sounds around you? Are they harsh? Do they frighten you? Are you hearing anything that is disturbing to you? Are you hearing things you know are not there?" Observation.

0 not present
1 very mild harshness or ability to frighten
2 mild harshness or ability to frighten
3 moderate harshness or ability to frighten
4 moderately severe hallucinations
5 severe hallucinations
6 extremely severe hallucinations
7 continuous hallucinations

PAROXYSMAL SWEATS – Observation.
0 no sweat visible
1 barely perceptible sweating, palms moist
2
3
4 beads of sweat obvious on forehead
5
6
7 drenching sweats

ANXIETY – Ask "Do you feel nervous?"
Observation.
0 no anxiety, at ease
1 mild anxious
2
3
4 moderately anxious, or guarded, so anxiety
   is inferred
5
6
7 equivalent to acute panic states as seen
   in severe delirium or acute schizophrenic
   reactions

AGITATION – Observation.
0 normal activity
1 somewhat more than normal activity
2
3
4 moderately fidgety and restless
5
6
7 paces back and forth during most of the
   interview, or constantly thrashes about

VISUAL DISTURBANCES – Ask "Does
the light appear to be too bright? Is its color
different? Does it hurt your eyes? Are you
seeing anything that is disturbing to you ? Are
you seeing things you know are not there?"
Observation.
0 not present
1 very mild sensitivity
2 mild sensitivity
3 moderate sensitivity
4 moderately severe hallucinations
5 severe hallucinations
6 extremely severe hallucinations
7 continuous hallucinations

HEADACHE, FULLNESS IN HEAD – Ask
"Does your head feel different? Does it feel like
there is a band around your head?" Do not rate
for dizziness or lightheadedness. Otherwise,
rate severity.
0 not present
1 very mild
2 mild
3 moderate
4 moderately severe
5 severe
6 very severe
7 extremely severe

**ORIENTATION AND CLOUDING OF
SENSORIUM** – Ask
"What day is this? Where are you? Who am I?"
0 oriented and can do serial additions
1 cannot do serial additions or is uncertain
   about date
2 disoriented for date by no more than 2
   calendar days
3 disoriented for date by more than 2 calendar
   days
4 disoriented for place/or person

Total **CIWA-Ar** Score____
Rater's Initials ——
Maximum Possible Score 67

The **CIWA-Ar** is not copyrighted and may be reproduced freely. This assessment for monitoring
withdrawal symptoms requires approximately 5 minutes to administer. The maximum score is
67 (see instrument). Patients scoring less than 10 do not usually need additional medication for
withdrawal.

Sullivan, J.T.; Sykora, K.; Schneiderman, J.; Naranjo, C.A.; and Sellers, E.M. Assessment of alcohol
withdrawal: the revised Clinical Institute Withdrawal Assessment for Alcohol scale (**CIWA-Ar**).
British Journal of Addiction 1989;**84**:1353–1357.

APPENDIX C
CLINICAL OPIATE WITHDRAWAL SCALE

Patient's Name:_____

Date and Time: _____/_____/_____

Resting pulse rate:____beats/minute
Measured after patient is sitting or lying for one minute
  0 pulse rate 80 or below
  1 pulse rate 81–100
  2 pulse rate 101–120
  4 pulse rate greater than 120

Sweating: *Over past 1/2 hour not accounted for by room temperature or patient activity*
  0 no report of chills or flushing
  1 subjective report of chills or flushing
  2 flushed or observable moistness on face
  3 beads of sweat on brow or face
  4 sweat streaming off face

Restlessness: *Observation during assessment*
  0 able to sit still
  1 reports difficulty sitting still, but is able to do so
  3 frequent shifting or extraneous movements of legs/arms
  5 unable to sit still for more than a few seconds

Pupil size:
  0 pupils pinned or normal size for room light
  1 pupils possibly larger than normal for room light
  2 pupils moderately dilated
  5 pupils so dilated that only the rim of the iris is visible

Bone or joint aches: *If patient was having pain previously, only the additional component attributed to opiates withdrawal is scored*
  0 not present
  1 mild diffuse discomfort
  2 patient reports severe diffuse aching of joints/ muscles
  4 patient is rubbing joints or muscles and is unable to sit still because of discomfort

Runny nose or tearing: *Not accounted for by cold symptoms or allergies*
  0 not present
  1 nasal stuffiness or unusually moist eyes
  2 nose running or tearing
  4 nose constantly running or tears streaming down cheeks

GI upset: *Over last 1/2 hour*
  0 no GI symptoms
  1 stomach cramps
  2 nausea or loose stool
  3 vomiting or diarrhea
  5 multiple episodes of diarrhea or vomiting

Tremor: *Observation of outstretched hands*
  0 no tremor
  1 tremor can be felt, but not observed
  2 slight tremor observable
  4 gross tremor or muscle twitching

Yawning: *Observation during assessment*
  0 no yawning
  1 yawning once or twice during assessment
  2 yawning three or more times during assessment
  4 yawning several times/minute

Anxiety or irritability:
  0 none
  1 patient reports increasing irritability or anxiousness
  2 patient obviously irritable or anxious
  4 patient so irritable or anxious that participation in the assessment is difficult

Gooseflesh skin:
  0 skin is smooth
  3 piloerection of skin can be felt or hair standing up on arms
  5 prominent piloerection

Total score:_____
The total score is the sum of all 11 items
(5–12 = *mild*   13–24 = *moderate*   25–36 = *moderately* severe   >36 = *severe withdrawal*)

Initials of person completing assessment:_____

Wesson DR, Ling W. The Clinical Opiate Withdrawal Scale (COWS). *J Psychoactive Drugs* 2003;**35**(2):253–259.

APPENDIX D
ALCOHOL ASSESSMENT QUESTIONNAIRES: BRIEF MAST, CAGE AND AUDIT

Brief MAST

		YES	NO
Questions		(Score)	
1.	Do you feel you are a normal drinker?	0	2
2.	Do friends or relatives think you're a normal drinker?	0	2
3.	Have you ever attended a meeting of Alcoholics Anonymous?	5	0
4.	Have you ever lost boyfriends/girlfriends because of drinking?	2	0
5.	Have you ever got into trouble at work because of drinking?	2	0
6.	Have you ever neglected your obligations, your family or your work for more than 2 days in a row because you were drinking?	2	0
7.	Have you ever had DTs, severe shaking, heard voices or seen things that weren't there after heavy drinking?	2	0
8.	Have you ever gone to anyone for help about your drinking?	5	0
9.	Have you ever been in hospital because of drinking?	5	0
10.	Have you ever been arrested for drunk driving or driving after drinking?	2	0

The Brief MAST is useful as a quick screening instrument to distinguish between alcohol-dependent (a score of ≥6) and non-alcohol-dependent individuals.

Pokorny AD, Miller BA, Kaplan HB. The Brief MAST: A shortened version of the Michigan Alcoholism Screening Test. *Am J Psychiatry* 1972;**129**:342–345.

The CAGE Questionnaire

1. Have you ever felt you should **C**ut down on your drinking?
2. Have people **A**nnoyed you by criticising your drinking?
3. Have you ever felt bad or **G**uilty about your drinking?
4. Have you ever had a drink first thing in the morning to steady your nerves, or to get rid of a hangover (**E**ye-opener)?

Two or more positive responses are a sensitive indicator of alcohol dependence.

Mayfield D, McLeod G, Hall P. The CAGE Questionnaire: validation of a new alcoholism screening instrument. *Am J Psychiatry* 1974;**131**:1121–1123.

The AUDIT Questionnaire

Circle the number that comes closest to the patient's answer.

1. How often do you have a drink containing alcohol?
    (0) NEVER   (1) MONTHLY OR LESS
    (2) TWO TO FOUR TIMES A MONTH
    (3) TWO TO THREE TIMES A WEEK
    (4) FOUR OR MORE TIMES A WEEK

2. How many drinks containing alcohol do you have on a typical day when you are drinking?
    (CODE NUMBER OF STANDARD DRINKS)
    (0) 1 OR 2 (1) 3 OR 4 (2) 5 OR 6 (3) 7 OR 8 (4) 10 OR MORE

3. How often do you have six or more drinks on one occasion?
    (0) NEVER   (1) LESS THAN MONTHLY   (2) MONTHLY
    (3) WEEKLY   (4) DAILY OR ALMOST DAILY

4. How often during the last year have you found that you were not able to stop drinking once you had started?
    (0) NEVER   (1) LESS THAN MONTHLY (2) MONTHLY
    (3) WEEKLY   (4) DAILY OR ALMOST DAILY

5. How often during the last year have you failed to do what was normally expected from you because of drinking?

(0) NEVER   (1) LESSTHANMONTHLY   (2) MONTHLY

(3) WEEKLY   (4) DAILY OR ALMOST DAILY

6. How often during the last year have you needed a first drink in the morning to get yourself going after a heavy drinking session?

(0) NEVER   (1) LESSTHANMONTHLY   (2) MONTHLY

(3) WEEKLY   (4) DAILY OR ALMOST DAILY

7. How often during the last year have you had a feeling of guilt or remorse after drinking?

(0) NEVER   (1) LESSTHANMONTHLY   (2) MONTHLY

(3) WEEKLY   (4) DAILY OR ALMOST DAILY

8. How often during the last year have you been unable to remember what happened the night before because you had been drinking?

(0) NEVER   (1) LESSTHANMONTHLY   (2) MONTHLY

(3) WEEKLY   (4) DAILY OR ALMOST DAILY

9. Have you or has someone else been injured as a result of your drinking?

(0) NO   (2) YES, BUT NOT IN THE LAST YEAR

(4) YES, DURING THE LAST YEAR

10. Has a relative or friend or a doctor or other health worker been concerned about your drinking or suggested you cut down?

(0) NO   (2) YES, BUT NOT IN THE LAST YEAR

(4) YES, DURING THE LAST YEAR

* In determining the response categories it has been assumed that one 'drink' contains 10 g alcohol. In countries where the alcohol content of a standard drink differs by more than 25% from 10 g, the response category should be modified accordingly.

Record sum of individual item scores here ____

A score of 8 produces the highest sensitivity; a score of ≥ 10 results in higher specificity. In general high scores on the first three items, in the absence of elevated scores on the remaining items, suggest hazardous alcohol use. Elevated scores on items 4–6 imply the emergence of alcohol dependence. High scores on the remaining items suggest harmful alcohol use.

Babor TF, Ramon de la Fuente J, Saunders J, Grant M., 1992. *AUDIT The Alcohol Use Disorders Identification Test: Guidelines for Use in Primary Health Care.* Geneva: World Health Organization.

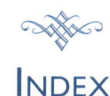

INDEX